American Academy of Orthopaedic Surgeons
6300 North River Road
Rosemont, IL 60018
1-800-626-6726

Revision Total Hip Arthroplasty

EDITED BY
WAYNE G. PAPROSKY, MD, FACS
Associate Professor
Rush Medical College
Chicago, Illinois

CONTRIBUTORS
John Antoniou, MD, PhD
Nelson Greidanus, MD, MPH

SERIES EDITOR
Thomas R. Johnson, MD

The American Academy of Orthopaedic Surgeons Monograph Series is dedicated to Wendy O. Schmidt, American Academy of Orthopaedic Surgeons senior medical editor, 1987-1991.

The Academy has made the material presented in *Revision Total Hip Arthroplasty* available for educational purposes only. This material is not intended to present the only, or necessarily best, methods or procedures for the medical situations discussed, but rather is intended to represent an approach, view, statement, or opinion of the author(s) or producer(s), which may be helpful to others who face similar situations.

Some drugs or medical devices demonstrated in Academy courses or described in Academy print or electronic publications have not been cleared by the Food and Drug Administration (FDA) or have been cleared for specific uses only. The FDA has stated that it is the responsibility of the physician to determine the FDA clearance status of each drug or device he or she wishes to use in clinical practice.

Furthermore, any statements about commercial products are solely the opinion of the author(s) and do not represent an Academy endorsement or evaluation of these products. These statements may not be used in advertising or for any commercial purpose.

ISBN 0-89203-242-1

CONTENTS

CONTRIBUTORS

John Antoniou, MD, PhD
Assistant Professor
Division of Orthopaedic Surgery
McGill University
Montreal, Quebec, Canada

Nelson Greidanus, MD, MPH
Assistant Professor
Department of Orthopaedic Surgery
University of British Columbia
Vancouver, British Columbia, Canada

PREFACE

Revision total hip arthroplasty is a complex procedure made up of a series of events that help determine the future well-being and function of a patient. The surgeon, faced with this complexity, may suddenly become overwhelmed. Many detailed textbooks have been written on this very complex subject. These texts, although very thorough, are often filled with a staggering amount of information that cloud many of the important reconstruction issues.

The primary purpose of this monograph is to provide a simplified femoral and acetabular defect classification system that enables the surgeon to determine the degree of difficulty he or she is comfortable in managing. In addition, this monograph renders methods of reconstruction for each type of defect based on ease of replication and rate of success at long-term follow-up. Alternative surgical approaches to each of the various defect types are also taken into consideration. It is hoped that the experience gained by one surgeon in performing revision total hip arthroplasty for nearly 20 years will help to make sense of a task that is often viewed as overwhelming.

WAYNE G. PAPROSKY, MD

INTRODUCTION AND ETIOLOGY OF FAILURE

NELSON GREIDANUS, MD, MPH

INTRODUCTION

It has been estimated that over 5 million artificial hips have been inserted since the advent of conventional total hip arthroplasty. Over 150,000 total hip arthroplasties per year are now perfomed in the United States, and over 10% of these procedures are revision arthroplasties. Recent statistics indicate that this figure is increasing as the United States' population continues to age.[1] Direct medical costs for all patient care currently exceed $15,000 per primary joint replacement, accounting for more than $1.2 billion annually. Revision arthroplasty is more technically demanding and costly than primary total hip arthroplasty, with expenses of $25,000 to $30,000 per case.[2] On the basis of these data the total direct hospital cost of revision arthroplasty is estimated to exceed $600 million, with increased morbidity and postoperative rehabilitation increasing total costs still further.

Using state-of-the-art techniques and materials, current arthroplasties are expected to remain functioning for 10 to 20 years. Most hip arthroplasties are done on older patients who are likely to retain their primary arthroplasties until the end of their lives. However, increasing numbers of young patients are undergoing hip arthroplasty, and the life expectancy of seniors continues to increase. Considering the finite life span of prosthetic components, in the future there undoubtedly will be an increasing number of revision total hip arthroplasties and an increasing number of patients returning for multiple revision procedures.

Successful revision total hip arthroplasty relies on many of the principles of primary hip arthroplasty but also demands additional attention to potential problems such as removal of failed components and cement, deficient host bone stock, and reinsertion of new components. Preoperative planning is of paramount importance as is knowledge of extensile surgical exposures, techniques of bone grafting, and understanding of revision component indications and insertion techniques.

In addition to understanding the fundamentals of diagnosis and treatment of the failed hip arthroplasty, the surgeon must be aware of the etiology of failure of hip arthroplasty components. Although improvements continue to diminish the failure rate of total hip arthroplasty, the surgeon continues to be challenged with failure due to materials, prosthetic design, technique, biology, and surgical complications.

ETIOLOGY OF FAILURE

ASEPTIC LOOSENING

Aseptic loosening remains the leading cause of failure in almost 90%[3] of revision total hip arthroplasties. National databases, such as the European hip registries, reveal that it has been the reason for revision in 79% of cases in Sweden, 87% of cases in Norway, and 83% in Finland.[4] Loosening rates vary depending on patient, implant, environment, and technical factors.

PATIENT-RELATED FACTORS

Survival analysis of hip arthroplasties indicates significant differences among age, gender, and diagnostic groups.[4] Among patients with osteoarthritis, men are at greater risk for requiring revision than women. Factors related to implant loading could explain the difference. Younger and more active patients also have a higher revision rate, as do obese patients, whose failures likely are related to mechanical factors. Patients with inflammatory arthritis have higher revision rates, possibly as a result of insufficient bone quality, and patients with hip fracture and aseptic necrosis are at greater risk for failure.

ENVIRONMENTAL FACTORS AND SURGICAL TECHNIQUE

Improved instrumentation, surgical techniques, and preventive measures to reduce the perioperative infection rate have been very effective in minimizing arthroplasty failures caused by septic and technical problems. Perioperative antibiotics, improved air ventilation, use of body exhaust suits, and use of antibiotic-containing cement have resulted in lowering infection rates to less than 1%.[5] Surgical and cementing techniques have been refined over the years with improved clinical results. The effectiveness of modern third-generation cementing techniques (pulsatile lavage, cement porosity reduction, and pressurization with cement plug and cement delivery gun) has been demonstrated in several studies, and these techniques currently are the standard for cemented hip arthroplasty.[6,7]

IMPLANT-RELATED FACTORS

Implant type remains important for success or failure of total hip arthroplasty. Decades of metallurgic research, hip simulator studies, clinical trials, and hip registry data have supplied information that can provide guidance in understanding implant failure. Well-designed implants have had low revision rates at minimum 10-year follow-up, whereas poorly designed stems have a tendency to premature failure.[8] In addition to design features, survival of metal components depends on appropriate metallurgic characteristics and biocompatibility. Improving femoral stem stiffness and fatigue strength with the use of forging superalloys has minimized rates of stem breakage. The use of corrosion-resistant and relatively biologically inert metals, such as stainless steel, cobalt-chromium, and titanium alloys, also has assisted in minimizing implant failures. The improvements in tapers and locking mechanisms in modular hip systems have further minimized fretting and corrosion as reasons for implant failure.

The original hip replacement implants consisted of two components, femoral and acetabular. Each of these components functioned as an articular surface, and fixation was provided through either cement or bone ingrowth. The introduction of modularity resulted in uncoupling of the surface-bearing demands and fixation demands of the implants. The advent of modularity provided further insight into the important qualities of each component in the total hip system. Improvements in both biologic fixation and cementing techniques have turned attention to the polyethylene articulating surface as the primary limiting factor in longevity of hip arthroplasty.

Minimizing wear debris and particle formation has become of primary importance in conventional hip arthroplasty systems. Debris and particles are now understood to initiate a host response to debris with recruitment of macrophages and subsequent osteoclast activation, which results in compromise of periprosthetic fixation and host bone. Particles can be generated not only by wear but also by fretting and fragmentation. However, the most common source of wear particles in hip arthroplasty continues to be the articulation between the femoral head and acetabular liner.

Although aseptic loosening and osteolysis historically have been considered separate processes, from a biologic standpoint they essentially are identical. The biologic process of aseptic loosening as it relates to the linear pattern of osteolysis that develops at the interface between implant and bone, whether that interface is metal or cement, is identical to that of the expansile, focal type of osteolysis that classically has been associated with cementless implants.[9] The difference is in the radiographic pattern of bone resorption determined by accessibility of joint fluid to the periprosthetic surfaces and accumulation of wear debris in the various interfaces. It is hoped that in sterilization methods and packaging and efforts to minimize backside wear will lead to reduction in sequelae related to wear debris and thereby to improved long-term results with the use of polyethylene acetabular liners.

Cemented Hip Failure

For most of cemented femoral stems, the weak link seems to be the cement-metal interface and the cement. Third-generation cementing techniques have improved the porosity, shear strength, and fatigue strength of cement. Texturing and precoating procedures have been used to improve the bond between cement and implant. There is evidence to suggest that long-lasting fixation can be attained and that creation of an intimate bond between cement, implant, and bone can seal off the interfaces from wear debris.[10] Once debonding occurs, there is increased access for wear products that can accelerate the failure of the hip implant. There is some suggestion that modern cementing techniques protect against lysis and loosening.[11] Despite improvements in the cementing technique, the long-term results on the acetabular side still are not as good as those for the femur. It is unclear to what extent the cement can protect the socket from biologic loosening caused by wear products.

Cementless Hip Failure

Intimate contact between implant and surrounding bone and rigid fixation are important to obtain bone ingrowth. Movement of more than 150 µm or a gap of 2 mm or more will preclude adequate bone ingrowth and favor fibrous tissue ingrowth.[12] Fibrous ingrowth components have an increased propensity to failure. Because the process of bone ingrowth is akin to fracture healing, indomethacin, diphosphonates, and radiation have all been found to decrease the amount of early fixation and the amount of bone ingrowth, thereby resulting in an increased propensity to failure.

Bone remodeling occurs more rapidly around cementless femoral stems and tends to be more pronounced than that occurring around cemented stems. Stem size, stiffness, geometry, and extent of porous coating appear to influence bone remodeling that features loss of density proximally with distal cortical hypertrophy.[13] This phenomenon of stress shielding classically has been ascribed to extensively coated cementless implants but is evident in most cementless and cemented stems. The resorption patterns seen on radiographs hardly ever have been reported as a cause for clinical failure, but they may indicate a more challenging revision arthroplasty in cases of compromised proximal bone. In proximally coated stems, gradual loss of fixation and radiographic signs of impending failure have been the major problems in both primary and revision hip arthroplasty.[14] An adequate, circumferential ingrowth surface appears necessary on both proximal and extensively coated implants to ensure reliable long-term fixation and to provide a circumferential seal to wear debris.

One of the forces behind the development of cementless technology was concern about endosteal bone loss, generally ascribed to the presence of acrylic cement. However, this complication can be seen with cementless implants as well. Implant motion and tissue reactions to metallic and polyethylene particulate and debris are the most likely mechanisms and can lead to the demise of the implant. The widespread use of modularity in cementless prostheses further increases the theoretical risk for debris formation from wear, abrasion, and corrosion.

REFERENCES

1. Graves EJ: Detailed diagnosis and procedures: National Hospital Discharge Survey, 1996. National Center for Health Statistics. *Vital Health Stat* 1998;13:138.
2. Barrack RL, Hoffman GJ, Tejeiro WVV, Carpenter LJ: Surgeon work input and risk in primary versus revision total joint arthroplasty. *J Arthroplasty* 1995;10:281-286.
3. Garino J: Etiology of failure, in Steinberg M (ed): *Revision Total Hip Arthroplasty*. New York, NY, Lippincott-Williams & Wilkins, 1999, pp 1-10.
4. Herberts P: Revision hip surgery, in Galante J (ed): *Total Hip Revision Surgery*. New York, NY, Raven Press, 1995, pp 1-17.
5. Lidwell O: Ultraclean air and antibiotics for prevention of postoperative infection. *Acta Orthop Scand* 1987;58:4-13.

6. Mulroy R: The effect of improved cementing techniques on component loosening in total hip replacement: An 11-year radiographic study. *J Bone Joint Surg* 1990;72B:757-760.

7. Barrack R: Improved cementing techniques and femoral component loosening in young patients with hip arthroplasty: A 12-year radiographic review. *J Bone Joint Surg* 1992;74B:385-389.

8. Malchau H: Prognosis of total hip replacement in Sweden: Follow-up of 92,675 operations performed 1978-1990. *Acta Orthop Scand* 1993: 64:497-506.

9. Maloney W: Osteolysis and aseptic loosening: Pathogenesis, in Steinberg M (ed): *Revision Total Hip Arthroplasty.* New York, NY, Lippincott Williams & Wilkins, 1999, pp 13-24.

10. Jasty M: Histomorphological studies of the long-term skeletal responses to well fixed cemented femoral components. *J Bone Joint Surg* 1990; 72A:1220-1229.

11. Schmalzried T: Hybrid total hip replacement: A 6.5-year follow-up study. *J Bone Joint Surg* 1993; 75B:608-615.

12. Callaghan JJ: The clinical results and basic science of total hip arthroplasty with porous-coated prostheses. *J Bone Joint Surg* 1993;75A:299-310.

13. Bobyn D: The effect of stem stiffness on femoral bone resorption after canine porous-coated total hip arthroplasty. *Clin Orthop* 1990;261:196-213.

14. Galante J: Clinical performances of ingrowth surfaces. *Clin Orthop* 1992;276:41-49.

EVALUATION OF THE PAINFUL TOTAL HIP ARTHROPLASTY

NELSON GREIDANUS, MD, MPH

INTRODUCTION

Appropriate standardized measures of outcome are essential in evaluating the results of total hip arthroplasty. Leaders in arthroplasty have long emphasized the importance of a standardized system of evaluation and have laid the groundwork for current clinical and radiographic measurement techniques.[1,2] Clinical measurements include description of pain, level of work and activity, walking capacity, patient satisfaction, and the results of physical examination.

A thorough history and physical examination are the most important elements of the assessment of a painful hip. In addition to obtaining a comprehensive orthopaedic history, the surgeon should seek to obtain a good general medical history. Items of particular relevance include those factors that could predispose to infection such as diabetes, inflammatory arthritis, disorders that compromise the immune system, history of prior hip infection, and multiple hip operations. Recent procedures such as dental work or invasive genitourinary or colorectal investigations or treatment may be relevant when considering septic etiologies for the hip symptomotology.

The location, temporal sequence, and characteristics of pain can provide important insights into the possible etiology of the hip symptoms. The presence of a pain-free interval after hip arthroplasty suggests implant failure or indolent infection as the etiology. Failure to achieve pain relief may suggest an extrinsic cause unrelated to the hip. Pain at rest and night pain suggest a septic etiology. The pain of aseptic loosening usually is aggravated with activity or weight bearing, with some relief with rest. Start-up pain in the thigh, which improves after taking several steps, often is described in the setting of aseptic femoral loosening. Groin or buttock pain may indicate acetabular loosening, and an acute onset of pain may indicate component failure, fracture, or hip dislocation. Heterotopic ossification may cause activity-related pain although rarely after the first few months of postoperative mobilization. Tendinitis may also give rise to activity-related pain but it usually can be localized well, and it responds well to conservative treatment modalities. Pain over the greater trochanter may be associated with trochanteric bursitis, iliotibial band tendinitis, nonunion of a trochanteric osteotomy, or irritation from hardware used to secure the trochanteric osteotomy.

The physical examination should include assessment of the lumbar spine and all major joints of the lower extremity and a thorough detailed neurovascular examination. The physical examination should include evaluation of gait, hip abductor function, limb-length discrepancy, and rotation. Range-of-motion testing may reveal contractures about the hip in addition to assisting in localizing the source of pain. Care should be taken to identify extrinsic causes of hip pain, which may include sciatic neuropathy, intervertebral disk pathology, lumbar spondylosis, degenerative spondylolisthesis, spinal stenosis, and vascular claudication. Other causes of pain in and around the hip include hernias and metabolic neuropathies.

DIAGNOSTIC EVALUATION

LABORATORY STUDIES

Once extrinsic causes of hip pathology are ruled out, tests should be used to assist in differentiating septic from nonseptic sources of hip pain. Laboratory studies are useful in the initial phase of investigation. A standard profile should include a complete blood count with differential and erythrocyte sedimentation rate (ESR) and/or C-reactive protein (CRP). The white blood count is generally of little value in the evaluation of the painful total hip. Leukocytosis is an uncommon manifestation unless there is acute sepsis. The ESR is a measure of inflammation. The ESR can be elevated as a result of pregnancy, connective tissue disorders, rheumatoid arthritis, malignancies, and chronic infection in addition to acute infection. The ESR can remain elevated for up to 6 months postoperatively and therefore is less reliable in predicting an infectious process soon after surgery. However, a value above 40 mm/h that persists more than 6 months after surgery is highly suggestive of an infectious process. The ESR has a sensitivity of 61% to 88% and a specificity of 79% to 100%.[3] The CRP is an acute phase reactant with normal levels of 5 to 10 mg/L. The advantage of the CRP is that it usually reaches maximum values 2 days after surgery and then returns to normal at 3 weeks. The CRP has a sensitivity of 91% to 96% and a specificity of 88% to 92%.[3]

RADIOGRAPHIC EVALUATION

Plain radiographs remain the standard method of prosthetic evaluation and can be useful in evaluation for osteolysis and loosening. An important part of the scheduled evaluation includes analysis and comparison of serial radiographs because subtle progression may be evident only when performing such comparisons.[4]

Gruen and associates[5] have classified lucencies at the cement-bone interface by designating roman numerals I through VII from lateral to medial on the anteroposterior view. Lucencies likely represent a continuum from solid fixation to gross loosening with increasing probability of loosening with increasing thickness and extent of the lucency. Lucencies along the acetabular component are described according to DeLee and Charnley.[6] The acetabulum is divided into thirds and designated with roman numerals I through III from lateral to medial (Fig. 1).

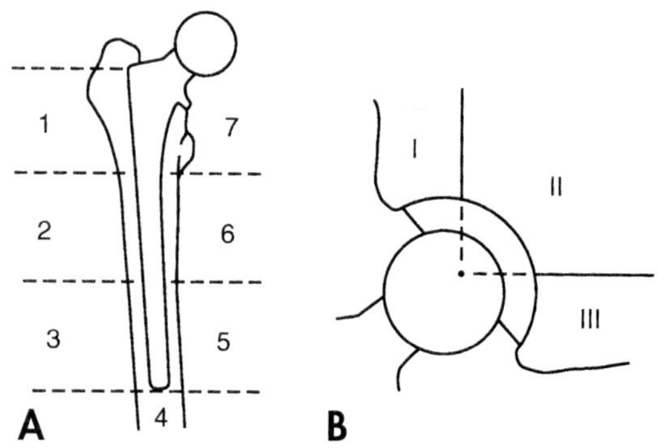

FIGURE 1
Classification of radiolucent zones. **A,** Gruen's seven zones of femoral lucency. **B,** DeLee and Charnley's acetabular zones of lucency. (Reproduced with permission from Schenk M, Dalinka MK: Radiographic evaluation, in Steinberg ME, Garino JP (eds): *Revision Total Hip Arthroplasty*. New York, NY, Lippincott-Williams & Wilkins, 1999, pp 121-140.)

Migration of the cemented femoral component is considered to be definite loosening. The amount of migration remains dependent on the quality of the radiographs and the measurement device used. Two to 5 mm have been suggested to be the lower limit for plain radiographs. Harris and associates[7] have further classified femoral fixation as possibly loose (radiolucent zone between 50% and 100% of the total bone-cement interface) or probably loose (complete radiolucency at bone-cement interface) depending on the extent of radiolucencies around the implants. Recent studies of mechanically stable femoral components have revealed that most cement-bone radiolucencies actually represent endosteal remodeling rather than disruption of implant fixation.[8] As a result, some no longer refer to the older femoral classification.[9]

Harris and McGann[10] also described two stages of acetabular loosening: definite (component migration or cement fracture) and impending (continuous 2-mm radiolucency). Hodgkinson and associates[11] have advanced current opinion of what constitutes cemented acetabular loosening. A 100% correlation was observed between radiographic acetabular migration and a loose acetabular component. This observation was confirmed by examination at the time of surgery. In addition, the acetabular component had a 94% probability of being loose when surrounded by a continuous radiolucency, a 74% probability when surrounded by a continuous radiolucency involving two thirds of the interface, and only a 7% probability with a radiolucency in only one zone. Therefore, socket migration of 2 to 5 mm or a continuous radiolucency around the socket are the current accepted definitions of cemented acetabular loosening.

Cementless implant loosening is more difficult to interpret. However, migration of the component by more than 2 mm is considered to be the definition for a loose implant. To further assist in understanding the radiographs of cementless stems Engh and associates[12] have described major and minor signs of fixation and stability. On the basis of these signs, they classify femoral component fixation as stable bone ingrowth, as stable fibrous ingrowth, or as unstable (Fig. 2).

Stable bone ingrowth prostheses have no demarcation lines adjacent to the porous-coated surface and endosteal hypertrophy (spot welds) at the junction of the smooth and porous-coated portions of the prostheses. Variable amounts of stress shielding are seen. If bone ingrowth has occurred, the implant is always stable. Stable fibrous fixation would result in parallel, nonprogressive demarcation lines adjacent to the ingrowth surface. In unstable prostheses, there is progressive migration of the femoral stem or progressive widening of demarcation lines around the prosthesis. There may be pedestal formation at the tip of the implant, hypertrophy of the calcar, or progressive bead shedding. Many of these signs appear to be component specific; radiographic evaluation of tapered titanium stems revealed minimal stress shielding and spot welds and cases of distal endosteal and periosteal cortical hypertrophy in clinically stable prostheses.[13]

The most reliable sign of loosening of either the acetabular or femoral component in cementless total hip arthroplasty is progressive subsidence, migration, or tilt on serial radiographs. Although some subsidence is not uncommon, it should stabilize at less than 1 cm and not progress beyond 1 year.[14]

The radiographs should be critically appraised for evidence of osteolysis. Osteolysis typically appears as a well-defined, focal lytic lesion that enlarges over time. Particle size, load, and composition and access of particles to the interfaces can affect the extent, location, and radiographic pattern of osteolysis. Expansile

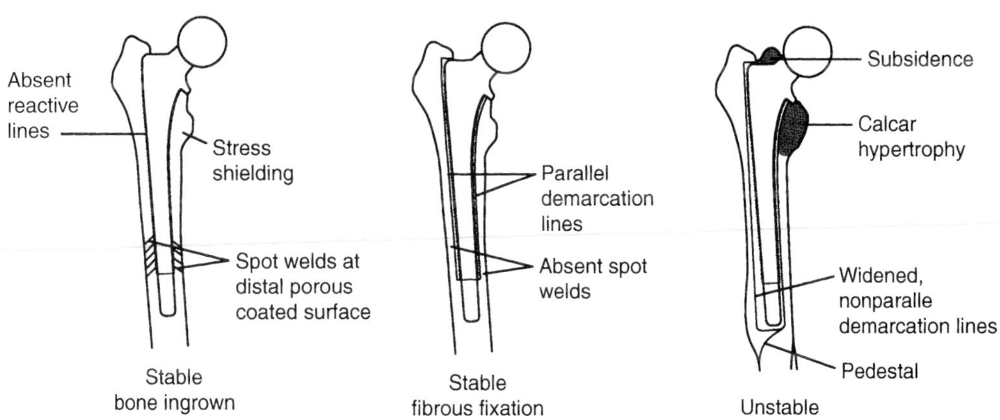

FIGURE 2
Engh's radiographic features of cementless stem stability and fixation. (Reproduced with permission from Schenk M, Dalinka MK: Radiographic evaluation, in Steinberg ME, Garino JP (eds): *Revision Total Hip Arthroplasty*. New York, NY, Lippincott-Williams & Wilkins, 1999, pp 121-140.)

osteolysis extending into adjacent cancellous bone may correlate with greater loss of host bone at the time of revision hip surgery. Although it often is asymptomatic, osteolysis may be associated with pain or wear-related synovitis of the hip. Osteolysis rarely is noted radiographically until 2 years after surgery; however, once detected it should be monitored at least annually. Rapidly progressive osteolysis remains an indication for revision surgery and further radiographic imaging by way of Judet views, or computed tomography scanning may be appropriate if the surgeon is concerned about major host bone damage.

Osteolysis often is associated with accelerated linear polyethylene wear (greater than 0.1 mm/y) that may correlate with factors such as patient weight and activity; femoral head diameter and material; acetabular polyethylene thickness, properties, and sterilization method; and system modularity.[15] Radiographic features of polyethylene wear include eccentric positioning of the femoral head in the acetabulum and narrowing of the superolateral margin of the acetabular polyethylene component. Metal particle accumulation in the region of the hip joint may indicate complete polyethylene failure.

Fractures of the sacrum or pubic rami may generate symptoms in the region of the hip and should be excluded as a source of pain from radiographic assessment. Bone scans or magnetic resonance imaging may be useful adjuncts in evaluating for fracture pathology.

ASPIRATION AND ARTHROGRAPHY

The overall accuracy of these techniques is lower than that of conventional radiography for both cemented and cementless hips. Accuracy of arthrography ranges from 51% to 92%, depending on the amount of pressure with which the contrast is injected, the presence or absence of pseudocapsules or bursae, and whether or not subtraction techniques are used.[16]

SCINTIGRAPHIC EVALUATION

As with arthrography, bone scanning is not needed in the routine evaluation of a painful total hip replacement, but may be performed when results of conventional radiography are inconclusive. In general, a normal scan provides more useful information than an abnormal scan, because it makes the diagnosis of loosening or infection unlikely.[17,18] However, a normal femoral implant can result in a positive scan in up to 9% of cemented stems at 1 year postoperatively and in cementless stems up to 2 years postoperatively.[19,20] An abnormal scan can represent loosening, infection, fracture, or heterotopic ossification. The situation can be further clarified with indium-111 leukocyte or Gallium-67 scans to increase the specificity for infection.

INFECTION

Infection must always be in the differential diagnosis of a symptomatic hip arthroplasty. This is discussed later in the section on management of the infected hip arthroplasty.

REFERENCES

1. Galante J: Editorial: The need for a standardized system evaluating results of total hip surgery. *J Bone Joint Surg* 1985;67A:511-512.
2. Johnston RC, Fitzgerald RH, Harris WH, Poss R, Muller ME, Sledge CB: Clinical and radiographic evaluation of total hip replacement: A standard system of terminology for reporting results. *J Bone Joint Surg* 1990;72A:159-160.
3. Spangehl M, Younger A, Masri B, Duncan C: Diagnosis of infection following total hip arthroplasty, in Cannon W (ed): *Instructional Course Lectures 47.* Rosemont, IL, American Academy of Orthopaedic Surgeons, 1998, pp 285-295.
4. Miniaci A, Bailey WH, Bourne RB, McLaren AC, Rorabeck CH: Analysis of radiolucide arthrograms, radiographic arthrograms, and sequential plain radiographs in the assessment of painful hip arthroplasty. *J Arthroplasty* 1990;5:143-149.
5. Gruen T, McNeice G, Amstutz H: "Modes of failure" of cemented stem-type femoral components: A radiographic analysis of loosening. *Clin Orthop* 1979;141:17-27.
6. DeLee J, Charnley J: Radiological demarcation of cemented sockets in total hip replacement. *Clin Orthop* 1976;121:20-32.

7. Harris WH, McCarthy JC, O'Neill DA: Femoral component loosening using contemporary techniques of femoral cement fixation. *J Bone Joint Surg* 1982;64A:1063-1067.

8. Maloney WJ, Jasty M, Burke DW, et al: Biomechanical and histologic investigation of cemented total hip arthroplasties: A study of autopsy-retrieved femurs after in vivo cycling. *Clin Orthop* 1989;249:129-140.

9. Schmalzried TP, Harris WH: Hybrid total hip replacement: A 6.5-year follow-up study. *J Bone Joint Surg* 1993;75B:608-615.

10. Harris W, McGann W: Loosening of the femoral component after use of the medullary-plug cementing techniques. *J Bone Joint Surg* 1986; 68A:1064-1066.

11. Hodgkinson JP, Shelley P, Wroblewski BM: The correlation between the roentgenographic appearance and operative findings at the bone-cement junction of the socket in Charnley lower friction arthroplasties. *Clin Orthop* 1988;228:105-109.

12. Engh CA, Massin P, Surthers K: Roengenographic assessment of the biologic fixation of porous-surfaced femoral components. *Clin Orthop* 1990; 257:107-128.

13. Mulliken B, Bourne R, Rorabeck C, Nayak N: A tapered titanium femoral stem inserted without cement in a total hip arthroplasty: Radiographic evaluation and stability. *J Bone Joint Surg* 1996;78A:1214-1225.

14. Kiss J, Murray DW, Turner-Smith AR, Bulstrode CJ: Roentgen stereophotogrammetric analysis for assessing migration of total hip replacement femoral components. *Proc Inst Mech Eng* 1995;209:169-175.

15. Jacobs J, Shanghag A, Glant T, Black J, Galante J: Wear debris in total joint replacements. *J Am Acad Orthop Surg* 1994;2:212-220.

16. Hendrix RW, Wixson RL, Rana NA, Rogers LF: Arthrography after total hip arthroplasty: A modified technique used in the diagnosis of pain. *Radiology* 1983;148:647-652.

17. Harris W, Barrack R: Developments in diagnosis of the painful total hip replacement. *Orthop Rev* 1993;22:439-447.

18. Lieberman J, Huo M, Schneider R, et al: Evaluation of painful hip arthroplasties. *J Bone Joint Surg* 1993;75B:475-478.

19. Oswald SG, Van Nostrand D, Savory CG, Anderson JH, Callaghan JJ: The acetabulum: A prospective study of three-phase bone and indium white blood cell scintigraphy following porous-coated hip arthroplasty. *J Nucl Med* 1990;31:274-280.

20. Utz J, Lull R, Galvin E: Asymptomatic total hip prosthesis: Natural history determined using Tc-99m MDP bone scans. *Radiology* 1986;161:509-512.

SURGICAL APPROACHES FOR REVISION HIP ARTHROPLASTY

NELSON GREIDANUS, MD, MPH

INTRODUCTION

Decision making regarding the selection of the surgical approach to the hip at the time of revision hip arthroplasty depends on many factors: the extent of exposure required and the anticipated pathology or magnitude of reconstruction (iliac, acetabular, femoral), the presence of prior incision scars, tissue and skin qualities, range of motion, limb-length discrepancy, comorbid neuromuscular conditions, and the surgeon's goals and familiarity with surgical anatomy. Basic surgical approaches commonly used in primary arthroplasty can be useful in limited revision arthroplasty procedures and include the direct lateral approach to the hip (Hardinge), the anterolateral approach (Watson-Jones), and the posterior approach. Extensive exposure often is required in revision arthroplasty and includes the trochanteric slide, the vastus slide, and the extended trochanteric osteotomy. The focus of this section will be on the use of the extensile exposures in the setting of revision total hip arthroplasty.

Several of the extensile approaches involve an osteotomy; however before performing such an osteotomy, the surgeon must consider both the extent of exposure needed and the bone quality of the patient's femur and greater trochanter. Osteopenia or osteolysis of the greater trochanter may jeopardize those osteotomies that involve the greater trochanter or predispose to fracture or failure of the osteotomy repair. Extension of the trochanteric osteotomy distally to include several inches of femoral shaft provides more bone surface for repair at the conclusion of the revision procedure.

THE TROCHANTERIC SLIDE

TECHNIQUE

The anterior trochanteric slide is an extensile modification of the lateral approach at the hip. The initial approach to the hip is the same as that for the lateral approach except that an anterior portion of the greater trochanter is osteotomized sufficiently to permit anterior reflection of the osteotomy together with the gluteus medius and vastus lateralis.[1] The osteotomy usually is made lateral to the insertion of the gluteus minimus; however, it can be performed to take the gluteus minimus with the osteotomy fragment. At the conclusion of the revision procedure, the fragment is reattached using cerclage wires that are placed through the osteotomized fragment and passed around the lesser trochanter (Figs. 1 and 2). The trochanteric fragment remains dynamized by the opposing forces of the gluteus medius and vastus lateralis, which contribute to its inherent stability. This osteotomy will permit reattachment and retensioning of the abductors to facilitate restoration of hip biomechanics and to assist in solving instability problems.

This osteotomy permits exposure of the femoral metaphysis to the level of the lesser trochanter, as well as improves exposure of the hip capsule and anterior acetabular rim. As a result, it has femoral indications that include the removal of well-fixed proximally porous-coated prosthesis and the removal of a failed monopolar fracture prosthesis with bone growth through its fenestrations[2] (Fig. 3). Acetabular indications include cases of acetabular protrusio that are not amenable to immediate dislocation and isolated acetabular revision procedures in which the femoral component is retained.

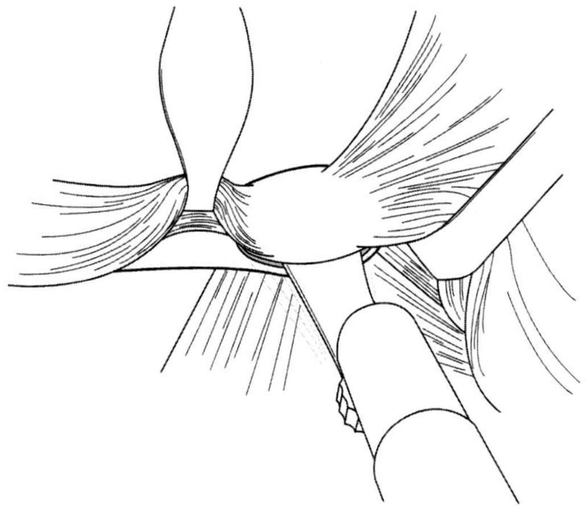

FIGURE 1
With the vastus lateralis exposed distally and the gluteus medius exposed proximally, the osteotomy includes their insertions and the lateral aspect of the greater trochanter. (Reproduced with permission from Engh C, McAuley J, Engh C: Surgical approaches for revision total hip replacment surgery: The anterior trochanteric slide and the extended conventional osteotomy, in Zuckerman JD (ed): *Instructional Course Lectures 48*. Rosemont, IL, American Academy of Orthopaedic Surgeons, 1999, pp 3-8.)

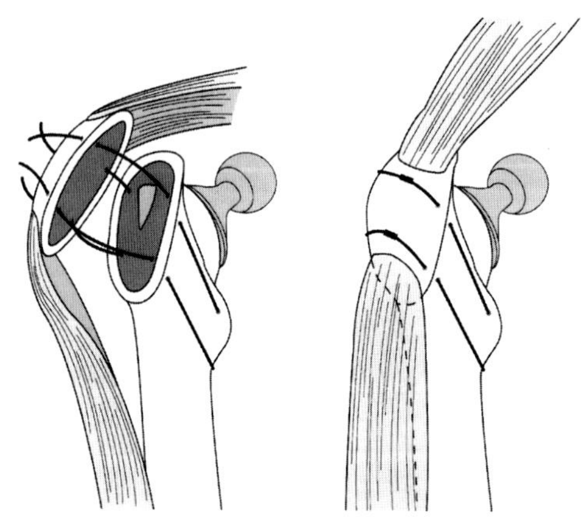

FIGURE 2
Wires are placed through or below the lesser trochanter and through holes in the greater trochanter. (Reproduced with permission from Engh C, McAuley J, Engh C: Surgical approaches for revision total hip replacment surgery: The anterior trochanteric slide and the extended conventional osteotomy, in Zuckerman JD (ed): *Instructional Course Lectures 48*. Rosemont, IL, American Academy of Orthopaedic Surgeons, 1999, pp 3-8.)

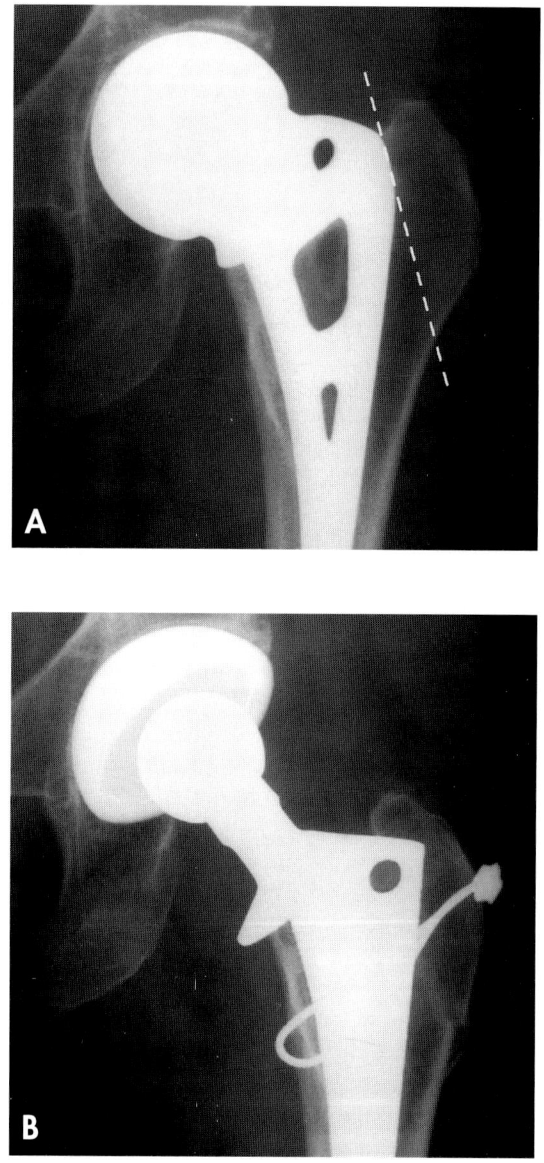

FIGURE 3
A, An anterior trochanteric slide will allow access to bone that has bridged the fenestrations of this implant. **B,** The osteotomy is repaired with a single wire or cable. (Reproduced with permission from Engh C, McAuley J, Engh C: Surgical approaches for revision total hip replacment surgery: The anterior trochanteric slide and the extended conventional osteotomy, in Zuckerman JD (ed): *Instructional Course Lectures 48*. Rosemont, IL, American Academy of Orthopaedic Surgeons, 1999, pp 3-8.)

POTENTIAL PROBLEMS

The small size of the fragment can make it prone to fracture, difficult fixation, or migration. In addition, if the revision of the acetabular component results in limb lengthening, the small fragment may not reach healthy femoral bone for reattachment.

THE VASTUS SLIDE

TECHNIQUE

The vastus slide is a variant of the lateral approach to the hip whereby the vastus lateralis dissection is extended to permit an extensile approach to the hip. The lateral intermuscular septum is preserved intact to minimize the likelihood of sciatic nerve injury. The slide technique is fashioned to appear as a question mark-shaped incision[3] (Figs. 4 and 5). The areas from A to B and the area from A to D in Figure 4 are exposed in a subperiosteal fashion. The subperiosteal dissection continues distally to gently elevate the vastus lateralis and vastus intermedius off of the femur. Care must be taken to ligate perforating vessels as the dissection proceeds. It is important to preserve a fascial cuff of vastus lateralis anterior to the intermuscular septum to permit repair of the anterior flap of tissues at closure. The proximal limb of the dissection is carried out to take only the anterior portion of the gluteus medius and minimus tendons. The surgeon must be careful not to violate the substance of the abductor muscle to avoid compromise of the superior gluteal neurovascular bundle, which passes through the abductor muscles 4 to 5 cm proximal to the greater trochanter.[4] An anterior capsulotomy can then be performed to facilitate dislocation. If further visualization of the femoral canal is required, the surgeon should consider an alternative extensile exposure or a proximal variation of the Smith-Peterson or Henry approach (Fig. 6).

Recently, an exposure has been described that utilizes the modified lateral/Hardinge approach superficially and then creates a posterior osseous flap, as in a modified extended trochanteric osteotomy, to facilitate cement removal or to address proximal femoral varus remodeling of the host femur.

POTENTIAL PROBLEMS

Neurovascular damage to the superior gluteal bundle with subsequent abductor compromise is rare, but it is an ever present risk with this

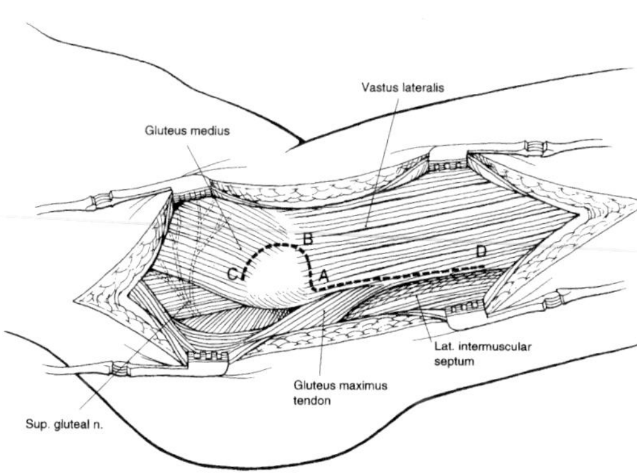

FIGURE 4
Vastus slide exposure. (Reproduced with permission from Head W, Montgomery W, Emerson R: Vastus slide and controlled perforations, in Zuckerman JD (ed): *Instructional Course Lectures 48*. Rosemont, IL, American Academy of Orthopaedic Surgeons, 1999, pp 13-17.)

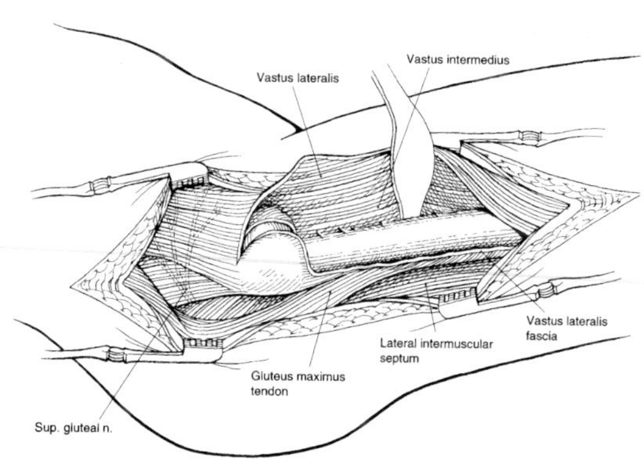

FIGURE 5
Reflected vastus slide. (Reproduced with permission from Head W, Montgomery W, Emerson R: Vastus slide and controlled perforations, in Zuckerman JD (ed): *Instructional Course Lectures 48*. Rosemont, IL, American Academy of Orthopaedic Surgeons, 1999, pp 13-17.)

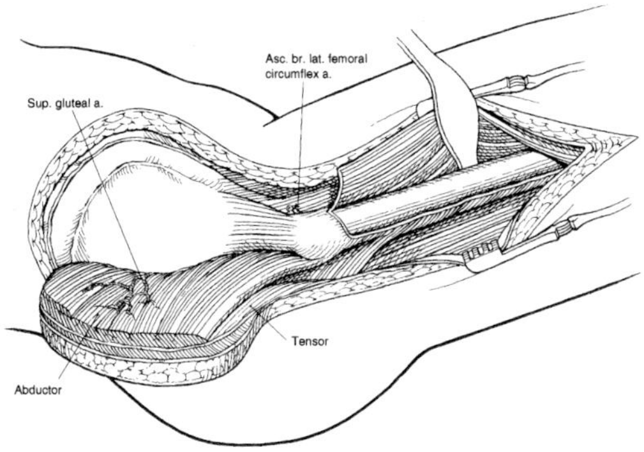

FIGURE 6
Deep incision, proximal extension of vastus slide to Smith-Peterson variation. (Reproduced with permission from Head W, Montgomery W, Emerson R: Vastus slide and controlled perforations, in Zuckerman JD (ed): *Instructional Course Lectures 48*. Rosemont, IL, American Academy of Orthopaedic Surgeons, 1999, pp 13-17.)

approach. Secure and anatomic repair of the soft-tissue dissection of the vastus lateralis and gluteus medius is necessary to avoid further potential compromise of abductor function. In addition, care should be taken during exposure to control the femoral vascular perforators to avoid risk of significant hemorrhage.

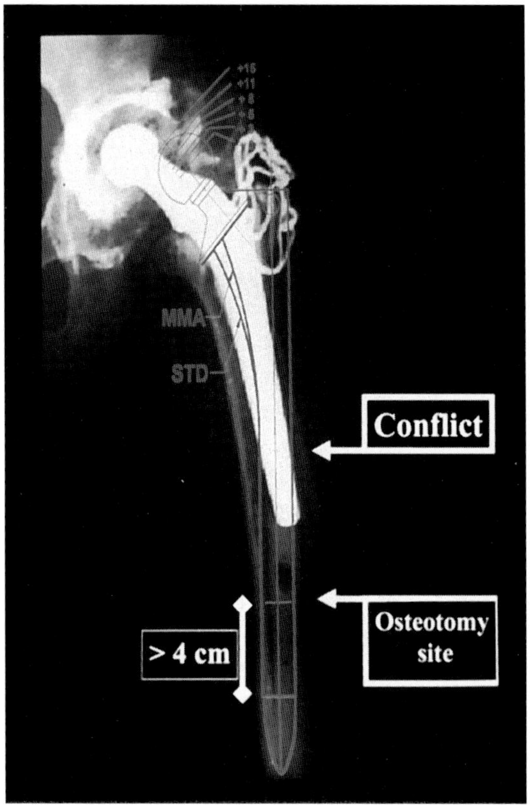

FIGURE 7
Varus remodeling of the proximal femur in a patient with aseptic loosening of the femoral component results in a "conflict," easily seen with a superimposed template. The site of the conflict and proposed osteotomy are marked. (Reproduced with permission from Arabindi M, Paprosky W, Nourbash P, Kronick J, Barba M: Extended proximal femoral osteotomy, in Zuckerman JD (ed): *Instructional Course Lectures 48*. Rosemont, IL, American Academy of Orthopaedic Surgeons, 1999, pp 19-26.)

EXTENDED PROXIMAL FEMORAL OSTEOTOMY

TECHNIQUE

This approach is an extension of the posterior approach to the hip that allows for controlled access to the femoral stem without devitalizing the osteotomized segment, which remains a viable myo-osseous flap. The osteotomy allows the abductors to be moved anterior as part of the myo-osseous flap, thereby further permiting excellent visualization of the entire acetabulum. This approach makes extensive acetabular grafting and implant fixation options possible in addition to having the advantages of facilitating correction of proximal femoral varus deformity. In cases of revision of cemented stems, the extended osteotomy hastens the time to complete cement removal without the need for femoral windows, and it has a lower rate of inadvertent femoral perforation or fracture. The extended osteotomy also hastens the removal of cementless stems.

Preoperative radiographs are templated to determine the length and diameter of the stem to be used in addition to the location for the osteotomy that will permit a minimum of 4 cm of scratch fit of the prosthesis in the femoral isthmus.

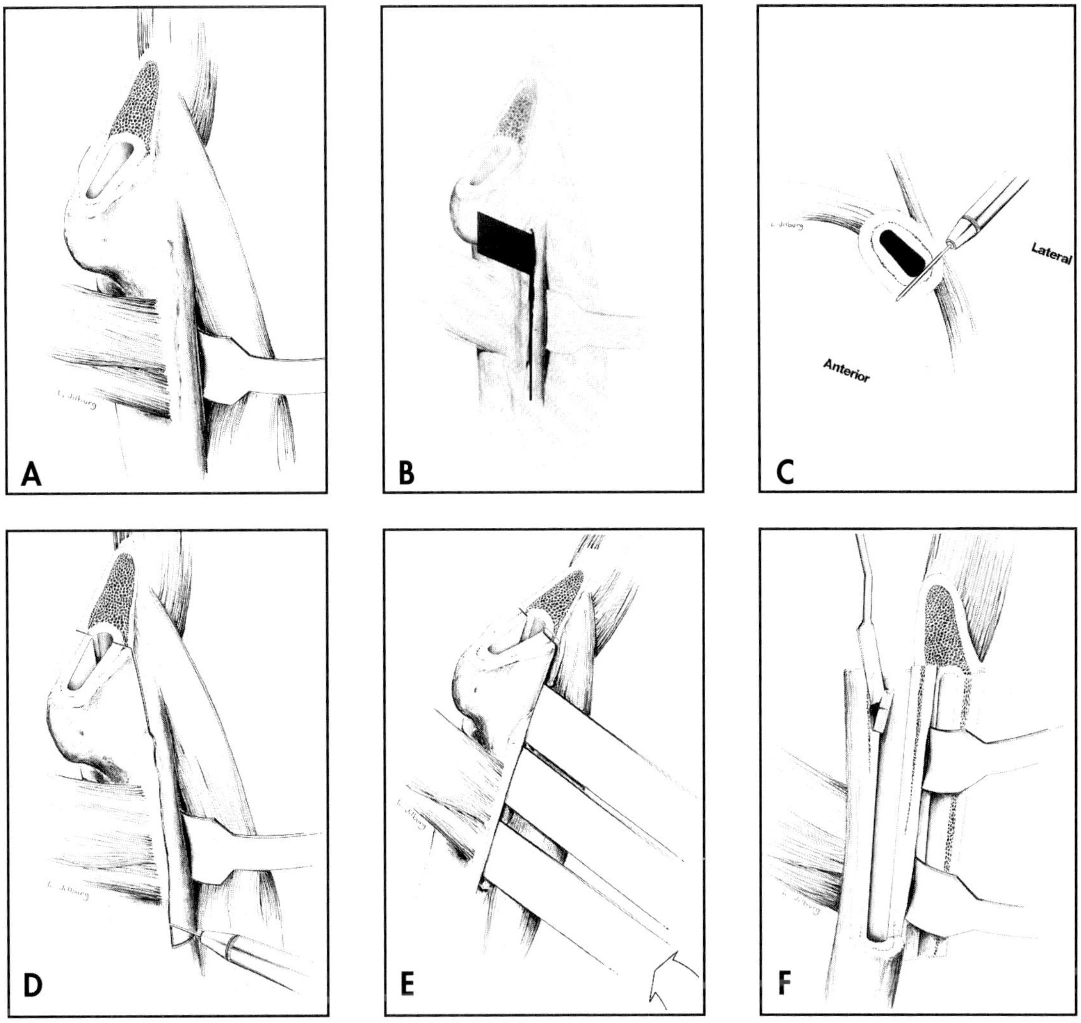

FIGURE 8
Surgical technique of the extended proximal femoral osteotomy. **A,** Posterolateral view of the femur, with a Bennet retractor holding the vastus lateralis anteriorly. **B,** After marking the osteotomy site, an oscillating saw is used to make the longitudinal limb of the osteotomy. The saw is oriented perpendicular to the anteversion of the hip. **C,** Cross section of the proximal femur. The saw is directed from posterolateral to anterolateral to perforate the anterior cortex. The osteotomized fragment should encompass the posterolateral third of the proximal femur. **D,** Proximally, at the level of the vastus tubercle, the osteotomy is angled medially to incorporate all of the greater trochanter. Distally, the transverse limb of the osteotomy is made with a pencil-tip burr to avoid stress risers. **E,** Wide Lambotte osteotomes are passed from posterior to anterior to gently lever open the osteotomy site, after the tight pseudocapsule from the anterior aspect of the greater trochanter is released. **F,** The osteotomy fragment is retracted anteriorly. The cement from the proximal femur is removed with offset osteotomes and high-speed burrs. The osteotomy allows direct access to the distal cement plug. (Figures *A* and *C* through *F* are reproduced with permission from Younger TI, Bradford MS, Magnus RE, Paprosky WG: Extended proximal femoral osteotomy: A new technique for femoral revision arthroplasty. *J Arthroplasty* 1995;10:3291-338. Figure *B* is reproduced with permission from Arabindi M, Paprosky W, Nourbash P, Kronick J, Barba M: Extended proximal femoral osteotomy, in Zuckerman JD (ed): *Instructional Course Lectures 48*. Rosemont, IL, American Academy of Orthopaedic Surgeons, 1999, pp 19-26.)

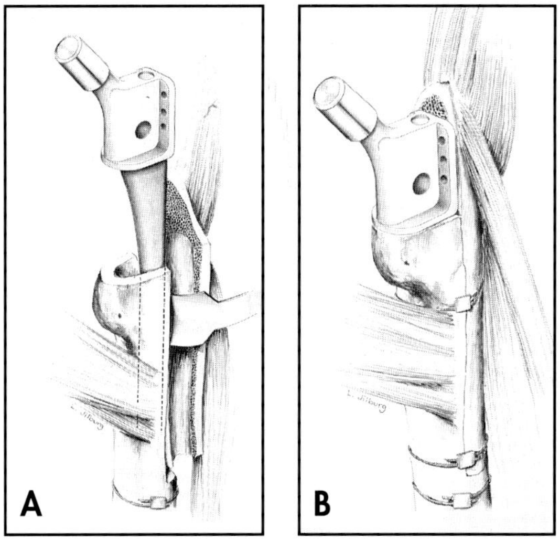

FIGURE 9

Implantation. **A**, Prophylactic cerclage wire is placed slightly distal to the distal extent of the osteotomy to prevent any propagation of fractures. **B,** On insertion of the prosthesis, cerclage wires are used to reapproximate the osteotomy site. Strut grafts may be added to augment fixation of the osteotomized fragment and supplement host bone. (Reproduced with permission from Arabindi M, Paprosky W, Nourbash P, Kronick J, Barba M: Extended proximal femoral osteotomy, in Zuckerman JD (ed): *Instructional Course Lectures 48*. Rosemont, IL, American Academy of Orthopaedic Surgeons, 1999, pp 19-26.)

Both the anteroposterior and lateral views should be evaluated with templates to determine if there are any potential areas of conflict for delivery of the femoral stems. Often varus remodeling of the proximal femoral around a failed varus femoral component can create such a conflict (Fig. 7). The extended proximal femoral osteotomy, which can be used to manage these conflicts, is essentially created as a compromise between access to the canal and preservation of fixation surface.

Following the incision of superficial dissection for a posterior approach to the hip, the short external rotators and hip capsule are raised as a single flap. Tthe gluteus maximus tendon is often then released to relieve tension on the soft tissues posteriorly and to appropriately mobilize the proximal femur. Following dislocation, the prosthesis is removed if loose, or the osteotomy can be done to facilitate removal. The vastus lateralis is then gently lifted from the posterolateral femur, and care is taken to ligate or cauterize vascular perforators encountered as the dissection proceeds (Fig. 8). The osteotomy site is then marked, and a pencil-tip burr is used to make the transverse cut of the distal aspect of the osteotomy site. Care is taken to round the edges so as to avoid creating a stress riser. An oscillating saw then is used to complete the posterior cut of the osteotomy including the entire greater trochanter. Wide Lambotte osteotomes are then used to elevate the osteotomized fragment anteriorly. This should constitute one third of the circumference of the proximal femur. The abductors and vastus lateralis remain attached to the bone fragment. Further release of the anterior pseudocapsule can prevent tethering of the osteotomized fragment and improve exposure. Components and cement then can be removed and reconstruction of femur or acetabulum begun. Before insertion of the cementless femoral prosthesis, a prophylactic cerclage wire is placed distal to the distal extent of the osteotomy to prevent any propagation of fracture (Fig. 9). Reattachment with two or three cables or wires can be performed once the components are inserted and stability is obtained. The osteotomized fragment can be reattached to allograft or repositioned to optimize hip biomechanics and stability. Arabindi and associates[5] report on 142 revisions with an extended osteotomy with no nonunions, malunions, or osteotomy migration and four osteotomy fragment fractures that healed without complication.

POTENTIAL PROBLEMS

Risks of fracture of the osteotomized fragment are present, and care should be taken to include a reasonable portion of cortical bone in the osteotomy to minimize this problem. As with all posterior approaches, a theoretical increased risk of dislocation and sciatic nerve injury exist.

REFERENCES

1. Masri B, Campbell DG, Garbuz D, Duncan CP: Seven specialized exposures for revision hip and knee replacement. *Orthop Clin North Am* 1998;29:229-240.
2. Engh CA Jr, McAuley JP, Engh C Sr: Surgical approaches for revision total hip replacment surgery: The anterior trochanteric slide and the extended conventional osteotomy, in Zuckerman JD (ed): *Instructional Course Lectures 48.* Rosemont, IL, American Academy of Orthopaedic Surgeons, 1999, pp 3-8.
3. Head WC, Montgomery WK, Emerson RH Jr: Vastus slide and controlled perforations, in Zuckerman JD (ed): *Instructional Course Lectures 48.* Rosemont, IL, American Academy of Orthopaedic Surgeons, 1999, pp 13-17.
4. Foster D, Hunter J: The direct lateral approach to the hip for arthroplasty: Advantages and complications. *Orthopedics* 1987;10:274-280.
5. Arabindi R, Paprosky W, Nourbash P, Kronick J, Barba M: Extended proximal femoral osteotomy, in Zuckerman JD (ed): *Instructional Course Lectures 48.* Rosemont, IL, American Academy of Orthopaedic Surgeons, 1999, pp 19-26.

COMPONENT REMOVAL IN REVISION HIP ARTHROPLASTY

NELSON GREIDANUS, MD, MPH

INTRODUCTION

Component and cement removal can be a time- and energy-consuming task for the surgeon undertaking revision hip arthroplasty. Many techniques and tools have been developed to facilitate this portion of the procedure; however, not every technique will be equally efficacious to every surgeon. It is important that the surgeon undertaking revision hip arthroplasty be familiar and comfortable with basic techniques to facilitate the most efficient and atraumatic removal of components without compromising fixation options for the revision components. Preoperative planning is of utmost importance, and regardless of the magnitude of the anticipated procedure the surgeon should always be prepared to encounter complications or the need for more extensive revision surgery than anticipated. The current hip arthroplasty components should be identified, old surgical reports obtained, and the appropriate company representative notified to verify the specifications of the component and to arrange for compatible componentry should there be a need to change only part of one component or only one component. Locking mechanisms, tapers, and removal equipment continue to evolve, and proper preparation will ensure that the surgeon has up-to-date information and components for the procedure at hand.

ACETABULAR COMPONENT REMOVAL

POLYETHYLENE LINER EXCHANGE

While this is considered technically the easiest of revision procedures, the surgeon must be aware of potential problems and pitfalls when exchanging the polyethylene liner. Preoperative planning must include verification of the current component with outer and inner diameter specifications in addition to knowledge of the locking mechanisms of the acetabular shell and polyethylene liner options. Although a cob or osteotome can be used to lever the liner out of the shell, this may damage the shell or locking mechanism. Many revision systems will have relatively atraumatic liner removal equipment available that can facilitate this procedure. One common approach is to gently drill through the center of the acetabular liner and then screw in a polyethylene insert extractor, which will gently lift out the liner. The surgeon should always be prepared to change more than just the liner and should consider the possible need to revise the femoral ball, stem, or socket if it is found to be loose or damaged at the time of surgery or if the hip remains unstable after liner exchange.

CEMENTED ACETABULAR COMPONENT REMOVAL

To effectively remove the acetabular component the bone-cement interface must be disrupted. Often the most atraumatic technique involves disrupting the cement-prosthesis interface first. The superior portion of the acetabular component should be exposed to enable the gentle passage of curved gouges and osteotomes to break the bond. Once this bond is broken, osteotomes, cobs, and curettes can facilitate the gentle removal of the remaining cement. Intrapelvic components or cement should be respected and assumed to be adherent to vital intrapelvic contents. Preoperative consultation with general or vascular surgeons should be considered, and further imaging or surgical exposures may be necessary in these cases.

CEMENTLESS ACETABULAR COMPONENT REMOVAL

Of primary importance in the removal of any cementless component is obtaining full exposure of the bone-implant interface circumferentially around the implant. Although this step is difficult at times, it likely will minimize the unknowing damage of significant host bone. A high-speed pencil-tip burr can then be used to develop this interface and allow for the subsequent passage of curved gouges. The surgeon must be careful not to lever the cup with the gouges because this may fracture the valuable host bone remaining. Once loosened, the cup can be grasped and removed. Another option, which exists when titanium shells need to be removed, involves cutting the shell into three quadrants with a metal-cutting high-speed burr. This technique is invaluable to the removal of medialized sockets. If this technique is chosen, the cup should be cut only after the periphery has been exposed and only after the host tissues are protected from the metallic fragments with saline-soaked sponges. After sectioning the cup, gouges can be used to gently free the component.

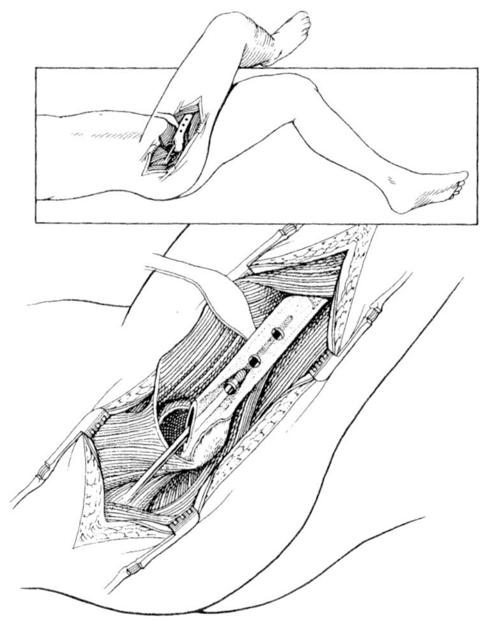

FIGURE 1
Controlled femoral perforations. (Reproduced with permission from Head W, Montgomery W, Emerson R: Vastus slide and controlled perforations, in Zuckerman JD (ed): *Instructional Course Lectures 48*. Rosemont, IL, American Academy of Orthopaedic Surgeons, 1999, pp 13-17.)

FEMORAL COMPONENT REMOVAL

CEMENTED FEMORAL COMPONENT REMOVAL

Removal of cemented femoral components requires disruption of the bone-cement and cement-bone interfaces. Before attempting removal of the component, care should be taken to remove any overhanging trochanter that may compromise removal or be fractured once removal is attempted. Once the proximal portion of the femoral component is visible and the shoulder cleared, a component extractor can be used to withdraw the implant. If the component is reasonably well fixed and a cementless femoral reconstruction is anticipated, an extended trochanteric osteotomy can be used to facilitate component and cement removal.

Cement removal may not always be necessary, and several authors describe recementing of a femoral component into the previous cement mantle.[1,2] Such situations include revisions for instability or limb-length inequality, isolated acetabular revisions in which femoral cement technique is adequate, or when the femoral component is removed without removal of the femoral cement mantle at the time of acetabular revision to facilitate acetabular reconstruction.[3] If cement must be removed it should be removed proximal to distal. Many hand tools have been developed to facilitate removal, and the surgeon should be familiar with the cement removal osteotomes, high-speed drills, and ultrasonic tools.[4,5] Occasionally portions of the cement mantle can be removed by screwing a tap into the mantle and providing an extractive force. Generally, the proximal cement should be split with osteotomes or removed with a high-speed burr where the bone is thin. Curved osteotomes and curettes can be used gently to free portions of the proximal cement. Once down to the cement plug, a drill can be used to create a central hole into which a

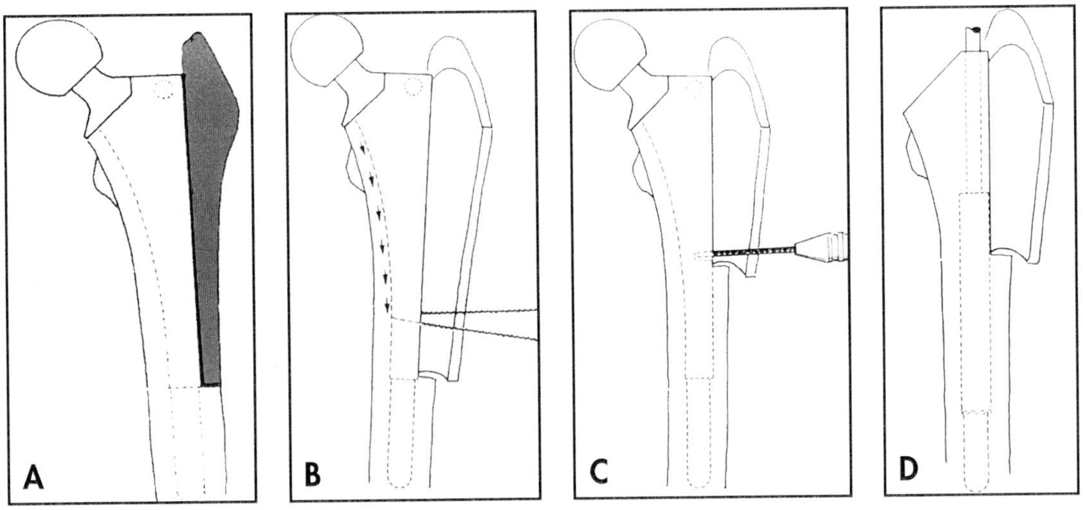

FIGURE 2
Extended proximal femoral osteotomy for cementless implants. **A,** The posterolateral cortex is sectioned as described above, but the anterior aspect of the osteotomy is completed by carefully levering on the wide osteotomes and creating a greenstick fracture anteriorly. **B,** The lateral surface of the stem is exposed and there is direct access to the anterior and posterior surfaces of the stem. A Gigli saw is passed around the medial aspect of the stem and directed distally. **C,** A metal-cutting burr is used to section the implant where its profile becomes cylindrical. **D,** Trephines are passes over the distal stem to remove it. (Reproduced with permission from Arabindi M, Paprosky W, Nourbash P, Kronick J, Barba M: Extended proximal femoral osteotomy, in Zuckerman JD (ed): *Instructional Course Lectures 48*. Rosemont, IL, American Academy of Orthopaedic Surgeons, 1999, pp 19-26.)

tap can be screwed and then tapped out. Adequate observation is necessary to avoid inadvertent perforation of the femoral shaft. Making windows in the femoral cortex proximal to the cement plug or obtaining intraoperative radiographs can minimize the likelihood of complications at this stage of the procedure (Fig. 1). If the drill and tap method is not successful, careful sequential drilling, burring, or reaming can enlarge the canal so that reverse hooks and osteotomes can complete the cement removal.

CEMENTLESS FEMORAL COMPONENT REMOVAL

Removal strategies should involve considerations as to how ingrown the component is, the extent of porous coating, and the geometry of the femoral stem. If the femoral component is loose, it readily may be extracted once the shoulder of the prosthesis is cleared of the trochanter. If the femoral component has bone ingrowth, special instruments and approaches must be used. In a well-ingrown proximally coated stem, use of cementless osteotomes and a pencil-tip burr may break the proximal bond sufficiently to allow a slap hammer extractor to remove the stem. In the case of a well-fixed, ingrown extensively coated femoral stem, an osteotomy may be necessary to remove the component. An extended trochanteric osteotomy, if performed distally to the junction of the tapered proximal body and cylindrical stem of the component, can greatly facilitate component removal (Fig. 2). Once the osteotomy is completed, passage of a Gigli saw around the proximal body of the stem can break the bond through the calcar region, thereby enabling the extractor to withdraw the stem. If the stem is fully ingrown distally as well, the stem can be transected with a metal-cutting burr, and a trephine can then be used over the distal stem to remove it while sparing the cortical bone of the isthmus.[6,7]

REFERENCES

1. Lieberman J, Moeckel B, Evans B, Salvati E, Ranawat C: Cement-within-cement revision hip arthroplasty. *J Bone Joint Surg* 1993;75B:869-871.
2. McCallum J, Hozack W: Recementing a femoral component into a stable cement mantle using ultrasonic tools. *Clin Orthop* 1995;319:232-237.
3. Hozack W: Component and cement removal, in Steinberg M (ed): *Revision Total Hip Arthroplasty*. New York, NY, Lippincott-Williams and Wilkins, 1999, pp 193-207.
4. Callaghan J, Elden S, Stranne S, Fulghum C, Seaker A, Myers B: Revision arthroplasty facilitated by ultrasonic tool cement removal. *J Arthroplasty* 1992;7:495-500.
5. Brooks A, Nelson C, Khofmann D: Minimal femoral cortical thickness necessary to prevent perforation by ultrasonic tools in joint revision surgery. *J Arthroplasty* 1995;10:359-362.
6. Younger T, Bradford M, Magnus R, Paprosky W: Removal of a well-fixed cementless femoral component with an extended proxiaml femoral osteotomy. *Contemp Orthop* 1995;30:375-380.
7. Glassman A, Engh C: The removal of porous-coated femoral hip stems. *Clin Orthop* 1992; 285:164-180.

ACETABULAR REVISION

NELSON GREIDANUS, MD, MPH

SURGICAL ANATOMY

The acetabulum can be divided into four regions: the superior rim (roof), anterior column, posterior column, and medial wall. The column description was first discussed in the context of acetabular trauma by Judet and associates.[1] The acetabulum can be considered as an inverted "Y," with the two limbs of the letter Y symbolizing the anterior and posterior columns. Radiographically, the columnar anatomy is portrayed as the iliopectineal line for the anterior column and the ilioischeal line for the posterior column. The iliopectineal line delineates the anterior column on both the anteroposterior (AP) and obturator oblique views. Disruption of the iliopectineal line indicates significant bone loss affecting the anterior column. The ilioischeal line delineates the posterior column on both the AP and iliac oblique views, and disruption of this line indicates compromise of the posterior column. Lucency that violates the iliopectineal and ilioischeal lines indicates pelvic columnar discontinuity or dissociation of the upper and lower portions of the pelvis.[2] The weight-bearing surface of the acetabulum is the roof or superior rim of the acetabulum, which is the junction between the anterior and posterior columns. The quadrilateral plate comprises the medial wall of the acetabulum, which is seen radiographically as the "teardrop" shadow.[3] The current classification schemes are based on these anatomic descriptions.

CLASSIFICATION

The most important role for a classification scheme of bone defects at the time of acetabular revision is to guide the surgeon to the best treatment option for the deficit that is encountered. In addition, a valid classification scheme enables the orthopaedic community to promote uniform measurement and reporting of surgical results. Over the past 15 years, several classification schemes have been developed. The most cited in the literature are the classification schemes of the American Academy of Orthopaedic Surgeons (AAOS) Committee on the Hip[4] (Table 1), Engh and Glassman[5] (Table 2), Gross and associates[6,7] (Table 3), and Paprosky and associates[8] (Table 4).

TABLE 1

THE AMERICAN ACADEMY OF ORTHOPAEDIC SURGEONS CLASSIFICATION SYSTEM FOR ACETABULAR DEFICIENCIES IN TOTAL HIP ARTHROPLASTY

Type	Defect
Type I	Segmental deficiencies
A	Peripheral
B	Medial
Type II	Cavitary deficiencies
A	Peripheral
B	Central
Type III	Combined deficiencies
Type IV	Pelvic discontinuity
Type V	Arthrodesis

(Reproduced with permission from Campbell DG, Masri BA, Garbuz DS, Duncan CP: Acetabular bone loss during revision total hip replacement: Preoperative investigation and planning, in Zuckerman JD (ed): *Instructional Course Lectures 48*. Rosemont, IL, American Academy of Orthopaedic Surgeons, 1999, pp 43-55.)

THE AAOS CLASSIFICATION SYSTEM

Bone defects are categorized as either segmental or cavitary. In type I defects, bone loss or segmental

TABLE 2

THE ENGH AND GLASSMAN CLASSIFICATION OF ACETABULAR BONE LOSS

Type	Bone Loss
Type I—Mild	Minimal–Both rim and cavity are intact
Type II—Moderate	Rim deficient, cavity intact
Type III—Severe*	Both rim and cavity deficient

*Protrusio acetabuli and pelvic discontinuity are subcategories of type III bone loss

(Reproduced with permission from Campbell DG, Masri BA, Garbuz DS, Duncan CP: Acetabular bone loss during revision total hip replacement: Preoperative investigation and planning, in Zuckerman JD (ed): *Instructional Course Lectures 48*. Rosemont, IL, American Academy of Orthopaedic Surgeons, 1999, pp 43-55.)

TABLE 3

THE GROSS CLASSIFICATION SYSTEM FOR ACETABULAR DEFICIENCIES IN TOTAL HIP ARTHROPLASTY

Type	Deficiency
Type I	Contained
Type II	Noncontained
Type IIA	Shelf/minor column < 50% of cup coverage
Type IIB	Major column > 50% loss of cup contact loss of 1 or both columns

(Reproduced with permission from Campbell DG, Masri BA, Garbuz DS, Duncan CP: Acetabular bone loss during revision total hip replacement: Preoperative investigation and planning, in Zuckerman JD (ed): *Instructional Course Lectures 48*. Rosemont, IL, American Academy of Orthopaedic Surgeons, 1999, pp 43-55.)

deficiency is defined as any complete loss of bone in the supporting hemispheric structure of the acetabulum. In type II, there is a cavitary deficiency in which there is a localized volumetric loss of bone with no disruption of the acetabular rim. In this classification scheme, the rim includes the medial wall. The deficiencies may be central or peripheral, and the peripheral deficiencies may further be classified as superior, anterior, or posterior. Central deficiencies indicate medial wall compromise. In type III defects, bone loss includes segmental and cavitary combinations. In type IV, bone loss describes situations of pelvic discontinuity or separation of the top and bottom portions of the hemipelvis. The fifth type of bony problem in the classification scheme (type V) refers to the fused hip because of the difficulties that can arise during reconstruction.

ENGH AND GLASSMAN CLASSIFICATION SYSTEM

This classification is a modification of the original AAOS classification. It contains of three categories. In type I, bone loss is minimal with the acetabular rim and cavity intact. In type II, the bone loss is moderate with deficient rim but intact cavity. In type III, the bone damage involves both rim and cavity. Protrusio acetabuli and pelvic discontinuity are subcategories of type III bone loss.

GROSS AND ASSOCIATES CLASSIFICATION SYSTEM

This classification is based on the nature of the bone graft needed for the reconstruction and whether or not there is 50% of host bone remaining. This simple classification has two types that can be classified on the basis of plain radiographs. However, the final decision regarding treatment depends on the intraoperative findings after the cement and membrane have been excised.

Type I represents those defects that are contained within the medial wall of the acetabulum and do not compromise the acetabular walls and columns. Medial wall deficiency may be considered contained as long as the acetabular rim and columns are intact and there is enough bone for the fixation of a cup or ring. Type IIA is an uncontained segmental defect (minor column) such that the structural bone loss affects a part of the acetabular rim and its associated wall or column totaling less than 50% of the acetabular contact surface. Type IIB is an uncontained segmental (major column) defect. It affects one or both columns and involves at least 50% of the acetabular contact surface.

PAPROSKY CLASSIFICATION SYSTEM

The use of specialized radiographs or computed tomography scans can be cumbersome and difficult to evaluate; therefore, this classification

TABLE 4

ACETABULAR DEFECT CLASSIFICATION

Defect Type	Superior Migration*	Ischial Lysis†	Medial Migration§	Teardrop Lysis¶
I	Insignificant	None	None	None
IIA	Insignificant	Mild	Grade I	Mild
IIB	Insignificant to significant	Mild	Grade II	Mild
IIC	Insignificant	Mild	Grade III	Moderate to severe
IIIA	Significant	Moderate	Grade II+ or III	Moderate
IIIA	Significant	Severe	Grade III+	Severe

*Insignificant = < 3 cm above superior transverse obturator line; Significant = > 3 cm above superior transverse obturator line

†Mild = 0 to 7 mm below superior transverse obturator line; Moderate = 7 to 14 mm below obturator line; Severe = > 15-mm lysis

§Grade I = lateral to Köhler's line; Grade II = migration to Köhler's line; Grade II+ = medial expansion of Köhler's line into pelvis; Grade III = migration into pelvis with violation of Köhler's line; Grade III+ = marked migration into pelvis

¶Mild = minimal loss of the lateral border; Moderate = complete loss of lateral border; Severe = loss of lateral and medial borders

system was developed based on information that can be obtained from an AP radiograph. The four criteria of hip center migration, degree of ischial lysis, presence of teardrop destruction, and extent of Köhler's line disruption are quantitated to determine the structural integrity of the acetabular walls and columns. This quantitation is the foundation of the classification scheme and appears to correlate with intraoperative bone defects and corresponding treatment options.[8,9]

Type I defects include those that do not compromise the integrity of the acetabular fossa. Bone loss is minimal with an intact acetabular rim and no major lysis or component migration. Type II defects include those that have moderate superior (< 2 cm) and/or medial migration without columnar compromise. The type II defects include three subtypes: type IIA is superior migration with an intact superior rim, type IIB is superior migration with superior rim compromise, and type IIC is medial wall compromise. The type I and II defects have at least 70% host bone remaining once the index component has been removed and preparation of the acetabulum has been completed. Morcellized or structural grafts are used only to augment host bone stock, and good fixation can be obtained using a cementless socket with screws.

The more severe acetabular defects are classified as type IIIA defects. A type III defect has more than 3 cm of superior migration as well as severe medial and ischial osteolysis. Therefore, the host acetabulum is unable to support an acetabular component at the anatomic hip center. Extensive bone grafting or the use of reconstructive rings is necessary to restore the hip to the anatomic hip center. While press-fitting a porous-coated implant is possible, it is difficult. The use of a structural allograft is recommended to reconstruct the deficient rim or column. Type IIIB defects are those with less than 50% host acetabular bone available to contact the acetabular component. Attempts to obtain fixation of the acetabular component with a porous-coated implant in such defects will be met with high failure rates.[8,10] For these type IIIB defects, it is accepted that there is not enough host bone to gain fixation of the implant to the host bone. An acetabular transplant allograft with or without a reconstruction ring is recommended to restore bone and provide a fixation point for the component to be inserted. These defects are the most severe and the most difficult to manage.[11]

MANAGEMENT OF ACETABULAR BONE DEFECTS

After radiographic assessment of bone deficiency, the degree of bone loss should be classified, and the answers to five important questions will direct the surgeon to appropriate management.[12]

1. Will stable fixation be obtained in the remaining host bone, with or without morcellized graft, so as to restore the center of rotation of the hip?
2. Are there segmental defects that will necessitate structural allograft, or will a high hip center be acceptable?
3. Is the bone loss so extensive that even with a structural graft, stability and fixation will be questionable?
4. Is there a pelvic discontinuity that will need reconstruction and fixation?
5. What is the optimal surgical exposure to facilitate acetabular reconstruction?

The opinions on managing acetabular bone defects vary from recommendations to avoid the use of bone graft whenever possible,[13] to recommendations to use morcellized bone only,[14] to recommendations to use complex structural grafts.[15] On occasion, bone stock must be restored because the extent of loss disfavors a high hip center or asymmetric cup. In addition, patients who are likely to need further revision operations would benefit from an improved bone stock for possible future surgery. Although rates of failure as high as 47% at 10 years after massive structural grafting have been reported, there are situations in which bulk allograft must be used.[16]

Bulk structural allograft can be anatomic (from a similar anatomic location) or simulated (from another part but shaped to fit the defect). In theory, an anatomic graft is structurally more able to withstand the biomechanical forces placed on it. For structural allografting of the acetabulum, some surgeons favor acetabular allografts because they are strong and can be sculpted to fit segmental defects in this area. They are fixed with cancellous bone screws, and if supporting more than 50% of the cup, they should be protected with a reconstruction ring.[17] Although structural grafts can restore the anatomy and provide structural support, they are susceptible to revascularization and remodeling, which can lead to resorption, collapse, or both. For this reason, if the anatomy and the limb length are acceptable without a structural graft, some surgeons favor placement of the cup at a higher hip center.[18] If a high hip center is used, the surgeon should avoid lateralization of the implant, and bone stock should be sufficient to allow the component to be seated against healthy host bone. In addition, the limb length issue must be resolved using a long-neck femoral component, and impingement must be avoided.

Morcellized bone (particles from 5 to 10 mm in diameter) can be used as filler scaffold in contained defects. Morcellized bone can revascularize and remodel and, therefore, strengthen over time.

COMPONENT SELECTION IN ACETABULAR REVISION

CEMENTED ACETABULAR REVISIONS

The early experience with acetabular revisions centered on the use of cemented polyethylene components. Similar to the findings with femoral revisions, there were high rates of mechanical loosening, ranging from 9% to 20%, with younger patients having up to a 41% re-revision rate.[19,20] Improved cementing techniques resulted in improved results, with mechanical failures approaching as low as 4%.[21] The results are affected profoundly by the quality of acetabular bone stock and cement mantle.

Cemented Acetabular Impaction Grafting

Sloof and associates[14] describe excellent clinical and radiographic results in 89% of 88 hips at a mean follow-up of 70 months. The technique of cementing an acetabular component into a bed of impacted cancellous bone remains a favored technique in many European centers.

Reconstruction Rings

Several studies have documented the outcomes of acetabular reconstructions using antiprotrusio rings. The technique involves fixation of a ring on a bed of host bone or a combination of host bone and allograft, with subsequent placement of a cemented acetabular component. The overall results of reconstruction ring procedures are less favorable than the results of other series largely as a result of the selection bias toward more complex cases. These patients often have the worst assortment of bone defects and, hence, have poorer outcomes. Rerevision rates range from 0% to 24% in the series in which such cases have been reported.[22-24] Increased infection rates are noted to be likely as a result of the increased surgical time, soft-tissue stripping, and insertion of hardware and allograft. Outcomes appear to vary depending on the magnitude of bone loss, the ability to obtain rigid fixation in both the ilium and ischium, and the ability to rest the majority of the cage on host bone.

CEMENTLESS ACETABULAR REVISIONS

Given the failures of cemented revision sockets and threaded cementless sockets, cementless hemispheric components have emerged with favorable results. Silverton and associates[25] report an 11% re-revision rate at 8.3 years with the failures not a result of aseptic loosening. Paprosky and Sekundiak[17] report no mechanical failure rate in patients with type I and type II Paprosky defects at a mean follow-up of 6.6 years in their series of 125 patients. Gross and associates[7] describe a 76% success rate with cementless sockets in conjunction with a structural graft for revision cases with segmental loss at mean follow-up of 7.1 years. Failures were due to aseptic loosening or graft resorption. Success appears to depend on obtaining good press fit of the component and rigidly fixating the sockets with screws. A minimum socket to host bone contact of 50% should be obtained to optimize biologic fixation.

Contained Cavitary Defects

Generally filling the cavitary defect with morcellized graft and reaming for a cementless socket will give good results, providing that screws are used to enhance initial fixation of the porous-coated device.[25] However, when there is less than 50% contact with host bone, the cup should be cemented to the allograft, and the allograft should be protected with an internal fixation device or reconstruction ring that extends from the ilium to the ischium.[7] Another option is to cement a socket into impacted bone.[14]

SEGMENTAL DEFICIENCIES

Medial wall deficiencies vary widely in magnitude. Some can largely be ignored and reconstructed with nonsupportive medial grafting if there is adequate peripheral fit during the acetabular trials. If there is insufficient peripheral stability at the time of trial fitting, the surgeon should be prepared to use a reconstruction ring to optimize fixation.

Superior deficiencies usually are apparent on the AP or the obturator oblique radiographs. Several options are available to reconstruct these defects, including acceptance of a high hip center, bulk allograft reconstruction such as number seven grafts or flying buttress grafts, impaction allografting, and customized components such as oblong cups. If the number seven or flying buttress grafts are used, distal femoral or femoral head allografts can be used, and rigid fixation should be obtained with two 4.5-mm cancellous bone screws[9] (Fig. 1).

Massive segmental deficiencies are the most severe bone deficiency states and should be recognized preoperatively and will show migration of greater than 3 cm because they may be technically demanding and unforgiving of improper reconstruction. Stabilization of discontinuities should be obtained using rigid internal fixation with pelvic reconstruction plates. In addition, a structural graft generally should be used to reconstruct the segmental defects using hemiacetabular or total acetabular allografts with restoration of the hip center of rotation. If less than 50% of the acetabular shell is in contact with host bone, then it should be cemented; if more than 50% of the shell rests on structural graft, the reconstruction would benefit from load sharing through a rigidly fixed reconstruction ring (Fig. 2). Some surgeons caution against using a reconstruction ring with morcellized graft alone to reconstruct a segmental defect because there may be a greater rate of ring failure by fatigue because the graft bed is unable to load share until the graft is consolidated.[7]

PELVIC DISCONTINUITY

Pelvic discontinuity has been described as an uncommon condition occurring in association with hip arthroplasty in which the hemipelvis is

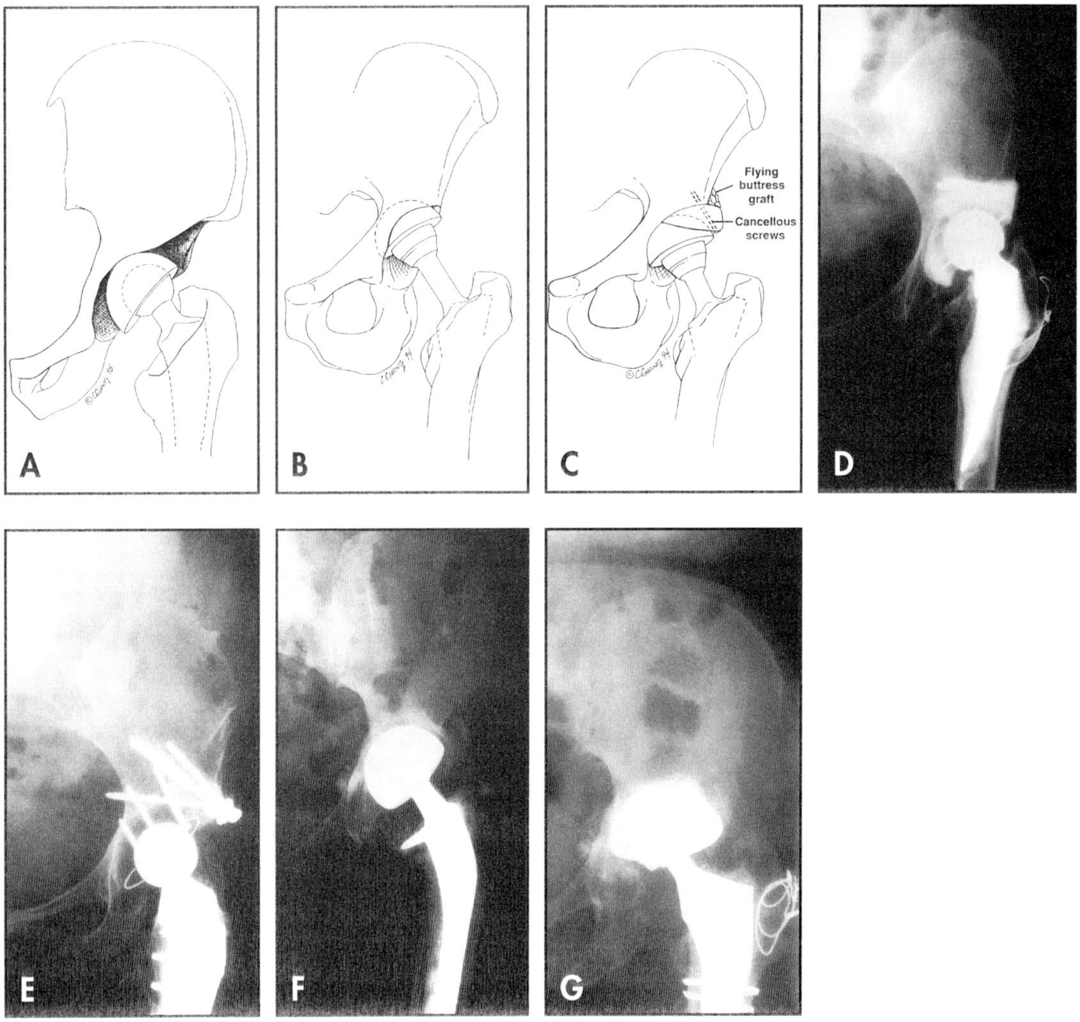

FIGURE 1
Structural minor column deficiency; Paprosky type II defect, Gross type II defect. **A,** Minor column defect (© C. Chang). **B,** High hip center with socket placed high to place cup completely against host bone in the management of the minor column defect (© C. Chang). **C,** A structural minor column allograft fixed by two screws (© C. Chang). **D,** Fifty-year-old woman with minor column defect 10 years after a cemented total hip arthroplasty. **E,** Nine years after revision arthroplasty with an uncemented cup and a minor column defect. **F,** Seventy-year-old woman 8 years after bipolar arthroplasty with a minor column defect. **G,** Seven years after revision with an uncemented cup placed high against host bone with no graft. Her bone stock was adequate and leg lengths not problematic. (Reproduced with permission from Garbuz D, Morsi E, Mohamed N, Gross AE: Classification and reconstruction in revision arthroplasty with bone stock deficiency. *Clin Orthop* 1996;323:98-107.)

separated superiorly and inferiorly by loss of host bone or a fracture line through the acetabular columns.[26] Berry and associates[26] have recently described 31 cases of pelvic discontinuity that were encountered in 3,505 acetabular revisions (0.9%) at the Mayo Clinic. Radiographic features of discontinuity may include: a visible fracture line through the pelvis or columnar lines, translation or rotation of the inferior hemipelvis relative to the superior hemipelvis, violation of Köhler's line, and superior migration of the center of rotation of the femoral head. Regardless of the presence or absence of radiographic features of discontinuity, it is imperative that the

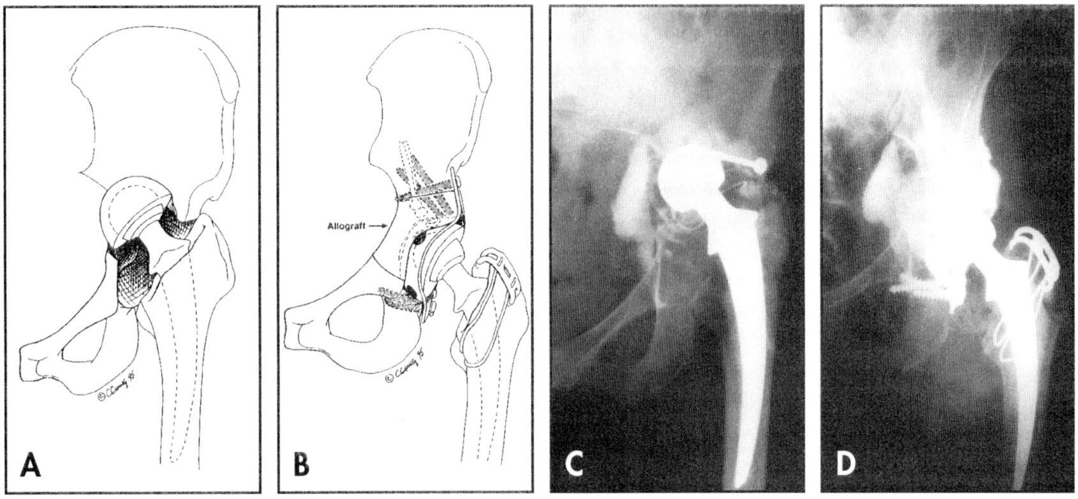

FIGURE 2
Type IIB Gross defect, type IIIB Paprosky defect. **A,** Segmental bone loss involving more than 50% of the acetabulum with a pelvic discontinuity. **B,** Reconstruction with major column allograft involving more than 50% of the acetabulum. The graft is held with two cancellous screws and protected by a reconstruction ring that goes from host bone (ilium) to host bone (ischium) (© C. Chang). **C,** Major column defect with perlvic discontinuity 10 years after cemented total hip replacement. **D,** Four years post revision arthroplasty with major column graft fixed with two cancellous screws and protected by reconstruction ring fixed to host ilium and ischium bridging the graft. (Reproduced with permission from Garbuz D, Morsi E, Mohamed N, Gross AE: Classification and reconstruction in revision arthroplasty with bone stock deficiency. *Clin Orthop* 1996;323:98-107.)

surgeon fully expose the acetabulum and verify columnar integrity prior to attempting fixation of the acetabular component. Berry and associates have proposed a discontinuity classification scheme based on the AAOS classification with type IVA representing discontinuity in the presence of cavitary defects, type IVB representing discontinuity in the presence of structural or combined defects, and type IVC representing discontinuity associated with previous irradiation of the pelvis. Excellent results were obtained in those cases with type IVA discontinuity while type IVB and IVC defects had less satisfying results with reduced likelihood of both discontinuity union and mechanical stability.

I have reported on 23 cases of pelvic discontinuity that were reconstructed at the time of revision hip arthroplasty.[27] The results were similar to those of Berry and associates with diminishing results proportionate to the magnitude of host bone compromise. As a result, we have proposed a classification scheme that identifies type IVA discontinuity as those cases with greater than 50% host acetabular bone remaining in contact with hemispherical acetabular trial components and type IVB as those cases with less than 50% host bone remaining.

A reasonable treatment algorithm for the management of pelvic discontinuity based on the above reported series would be: rigid plate fixation of the discontinuity followed by cementless socket fixation for cases with greater than 50% host bone remaining, rigid plate fixation and/or antiprotrusio cage placement plus allograft and cemented socket for those cases with less than 50% host bone remaining in the acetabulum. The ability of the antiprotrusio cage to load share while the discontinuity unites and the allograft incorporates appears to be invaluable to the successful reconstruction of the discontinuity with significant host bone loss.

POSTOPERATIVE MANAGEMENT

Patients with cementless socket reconstructions with contained cavitary defects are allowed to bear one third of their weight for 6 to 8 weeks and then proceed to full weight bearing. Patients with number seven graft reconstruction or flying buttress grafts are restricted to toe-touch weight bearing for 3 months and then one third weight bearing for an additional month. Patients then proceed to full weight bearing. Hemiacetabular and total acetabular graft recipients as well as pateints with pelvic discontinuity are restricted to toe-touch weight bearing for 3 months, followed by 3 months of one third weight bearing before full weight bearing. All patients are placed in a hip abduction orthosis to be worn when out of bed for the first 6 to 12 weeks. A knee-ankle-foot extension is often added for additional control in select individuals who display lack of muscle control postoperatively. All patients receive 24 hours of antibiotic prophylaxis with the exception of the acetabular transplants who receive 5 days of prophylaxis. Radiographic and clinical follow-up are at 2, 6, and 12 weeks after surgery, and then at 6 and 12 months, and yearly thereafter.

REFERENCES

1. Judet R, Judet J, Letournel E: Fractures of the acetabulum: Classification and surgical approaches for open reduction: Preliminary report. *J Bone Joint Surg* 1964:46A:1615-1646.
2. Masri B, Duncan C: Classification of bone loss in total hip arthroplasty, in Pritchard D (ed): *Instructional Course Lectures 45*. Rosemont, IL, American Academy of Orthopaedic Surgery, 1996, pp 199-208.
3. Bowerman J, Sena J, Chang R: The teardrop shadow of the pelvis: Anatomy and clinical significance. *Radiology* 1982;143:659-662.
4. D'Antonio J, Capello W, Borden L, et al: Classification and mangement of acetabular abnormalities in total hip arthroplasty. *Clin Orthop* 1989;243:126-137.
5. Engh C, Glassman A: Cementless revision of failed total hip replacement: An update, in Tullos HS (ed): *Instructional Course Lectures XL*. Park Ridge, IL, American Academy of Orthopaedic Surgeons, 1991, pp 189-197.
6. Gross A, Allan D, Catre M, et al: Bone grafts in hip replacement surgery: The pelvic side. *Orthop Clin North Am* 1993;24:679-695.
7. Gross AE, Duncan CP, Garbuz D, Mohamed EMZ: Revision arthroplasty of the acetabulum in association with loss of bone stock, in Zuckerman JD (ed): *Instructional Course Lectures 48*. Rosemont, IL, American Academy of Orthopaedic Surgeons, 1999, pp 57-66.
8. Paprosky W, Perona P, Lawrence J: Acetaular defect classification and surgical reconstruction in revision arthroplasty: A 6-year follow-up evaluation. *J Arthroplasty* 1994;9:33-44.
9. Paprosky W, Magnus R: Principles of bone grafting in revision total hip arthroplasty: Acetabular technique. *Clin Orthop* 1994;298:147-155.
10. Garbuz D, Morsi E, Gross A: Revision of the acetaular component of a total hip arthroplasty with a massive structural allograft: Study with a minimim five-year follow-up. *J Bone Joint Surg* 1996;78A:693-697.
11. Bradford M, Paprosky W: Total acetaular transplant allograft reconstruction of the severely deficient acetaulum. *Semin Arthroplasty* 1995; 6:86-95.
12. Campbell DG, Masri BA, Garbuz DS, Duncan CP: Acetabular bone loss during revision total hip replacement: preoperative investigation and planning, in Zuckerman JD (ed): *Instructional Course Lectures 48*. Rosemont, IL, American Academy of Orthopaedic Surgeons, 1999, pp 43-55.
13. Jasty M, Harris W: Salvage total hip reconstruction in patients with major acetabular bone deficiency using structural femoral head allografts. *J Bone Joint Surg* 1990;72B:63-67.
14. Sloof T, Schimmel J, Buma P: Cemented fixation with bone grafts. *Orthop Clin North Am* 1993;24:667-677.
15. Oakeshott R, Morgan D, Zukor D, Rudan J, Brooks P, Gross A: Revision total hip arthroplasty with osseous allograft reconstruction: A clinical and roentgenographic analysis. *Clin Orthop* 1987;225:37-61.
16. Kwong L, Jasty M, Harris W: High failure rate of bulk femoral head allografts in total hip acetabular reconstructions at 10 years. *J Arthroplasty* 1993;8:341-346.

17. Paprosky WG, Sekundiak TD: Total acetabular allografts, in Zuckerman JD (ed): *Instructional Course Lectures 48*. Rosemont, IL, American Academy of Orthopaedic Surgeons, 1999, pp 67-76.

18. Russotti G, Harris W: Proximal placement of the acetabular component in total hip arthroplasty: A long-term follow-up study. *J Bone Joint Surg* 1991;73A:587-592.

19. Mahomed N, Katz J: Revision total hip arthroplasty: Indications and outcomes. *Arthritis Rheum* 1996;39:1939-1950.

20. Stromberg C, Herberts P, Ahnfelt L: Revision total hip arthroplasty in patients younger than 55 years old: Clinical and radiologic results after 4 years. *J Arthroplasty* 1988;3:47-59.

21. Iorio R, Eftekhar N, Kobayashi S, Grelsamer RP: Cemented revision of failed total hip arthroplasty: Suvivorship analysis. *Clin Orthop* 1995;316:121-130.

22. Gill T, Sledge C, Muller M: The Burch-Schneider anti-protrusio cage in revision total hip arthroplasty: Indications, principles, and long-term results. *J Bone Joint Surg* 1998;80B:946-953.

23. Brady O, Masri B, Garbuz D, Duncan C: Use of reconstruction rings for the mangement of acetabular bone loss during revision hip surgery. *J Am Acad Orthop Surg* 1999;7:1-7.

24. Zehntner M, Ganz R: Midterm results (5.5-10 years) of acetabular allograft reconstruction with the acetabular reinforcement ring during total hip revision. *J Arthroplasty* 1994;9:469-479.

25. Silverton C, Rosenberg A, Sheinkop M, Kull L, Galante J: Revision of the acetabular component without cement after total hip arthroplasty: A follow-up note regarding results at seven to eleven years. *J Bone Joint Surg Am* 1996;78:1366-1370.

26. Berry D, Lewallen D, Hanssen A, Cabanella M: Pelvic discontinuity in revision total hip arthroplasty. *J Bone Joint Surg Am* 1999;81:1692-1702.

27. Greidanus N, Antoniou J, Paprosky W: Management of pelvic discontinuity in revision hip arthroplasty. Proceedings of the American Academy of Orthopaedic Surgeons Annual Meeting, Orlando, Florida. Rosemont, IL, American Academy of Orthopaedic Surgeons, 2000.

FEMORAL REVISION

JOHN ANTONIOU, MD, PhD

INTRODUCTION

The revision of loose femoral components can be a complex procedure for the reconstructive surgeon. The loss of femoral bone stock renders this problem a persistent challenge. The radiographic evaluation of loosening of cemented versus uncemented femoral components involves two distinct processes.

RADIOGRAPHIC EVALUATION OF FEMORAL COMPONENTS

The radiographic identification of loosened cemented femoral components can be divided into three categories as described by O'Neill and Harris.[1] A component is considered definitively loose with migration of the component and/or cement column, fracture and/or fragmentation of the cement, or fracture and/or deformation of the component (Fig. 1). A component is considered probably loose when there is a radiolucent zone at the cement-bone interface around the periphery of the entire component on at least one radiograph. A component is considered possibly loose when there is a radiolucent zone at the cement-bone interface, which extends for more than 50% but less than 100% of the periphery of the component. It is important to remember that these guidelines need to be correlated with clinical findings. Less than 2 mm subsidence of the femoral component does not affect the long-term result and is not a sign of loosening.

The radiographic identification of loosened uncemented femoral components has been elucidated by Engh and associates.[2] Evaluation of uncemented stems for loosening involves looking for the absence of bone ingrowth (Fig. 2). Signs of ingrowth include spot welds that occur at the distal limit of the porous coating, stress shielding of the proximal femur, lack of a distal pedestal, or lack of reactive lines around the porous-coated portion of the stem. Absence of these signs indicates that the stem is either fibrous stable or fibrous unstable. In a fibrous stable implant, signs of bone ingrowth are absent but there is a small distal pedestal, a radiolucent line around the circumference of the prosthesis that is less than 1-mm thick with reactive bone formation parallel to the prosthesis, a lack of proximal stress shielding, or slight calcar hypertrophy. In a fibrous unstable implant,

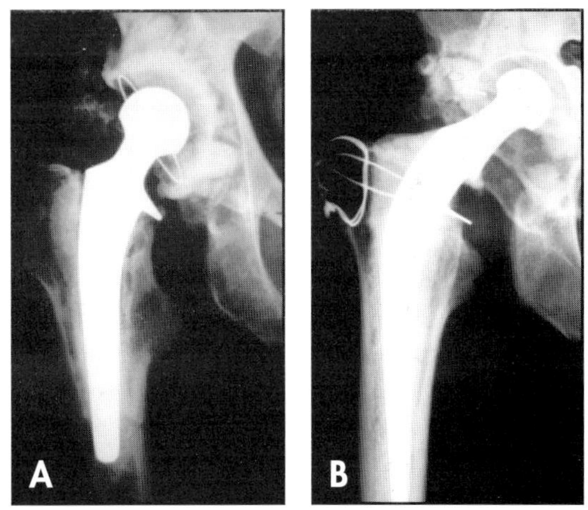

FIGURE 1
A, Asymmetric polyethylene wear with complete periacetabular radiolucency of cemented component with varus shift of femoral component and medial osteolysis. **B,** Severe polyethylene wear with protrusio acetabuli secondary to loose acetabular component.

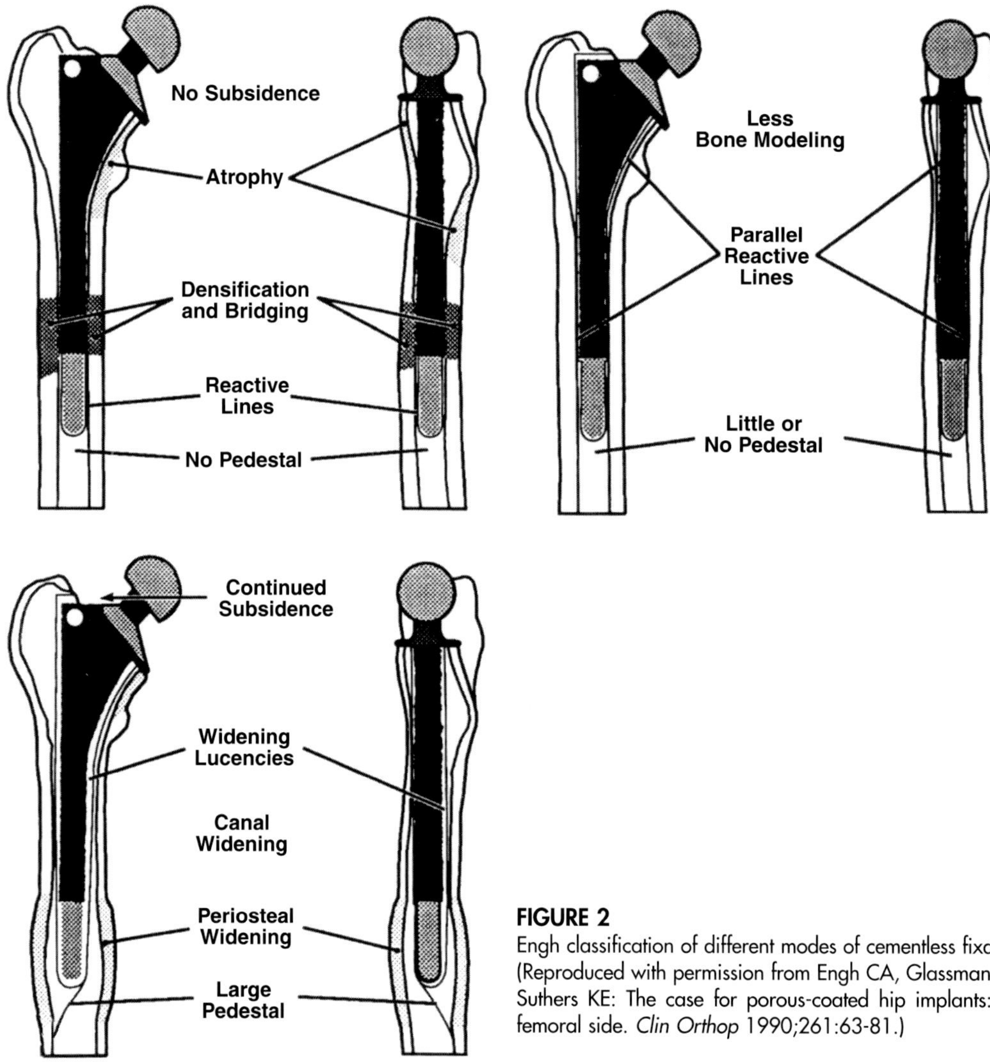

FIGURE 2
Engh classification of different modes of cementless fixation. (Reproduced with permission from Engh CA, Glassman AH, Suthers KE: The case for porous-coated hip implants: The femoral side. *Clin Orthop* 1990;261:63-81.)

signs of bone ingrowth are absent but there is a solid distal pedestal, calcar hypertrophy, reactive lines around the prosthesis that are divergent, or gross migration of the component.

CLASSIFICATION OF FEMORAL DEFECTS

A classification system is used to create a standardized method of describing and comparing femoral defects and to aid in the creation of treatment algorithms. Several classification systems for femoral bone loss have been described, although none of these systems has found widespread acceptance or been validated independently. Classification systems with varied complexity have been characterized by Chandler and Penenberg,[3] Dorr and associates,[4] Engh and Glassman,[5] Gross and associates,[6] Mallory,[7] and Paprosky and associates.[8]

THE AMERICAN ACADEMY OF ORTHOPAEDIC SURGEONS CLASSIFICATION SYSTEM

The American Academy of Othopaedic Surgeons (AAOS) has adapted a femoral classification system developed by D'Antonio and associates[9] that divides bone loss into segmental and cavitary defects. This system attempts to address bone deficiency in both the primary and revision settings. Segmental defects involve loss of bone in the cortical shell of the femur and are divided into partial and complete. Cavitary defects are either cancellous or endosteal cortical without violation of the outer shell. Combined defects have both segmental and cavitary bone loss.

This system also has a category for femoral alignment, stenosis, discontinuity, and the level of bone loss. Level 1 bone loss is proximal to the bottom of the lesser trochanter, level 2 is 10 cm distal to level 1, and level 3 is everything distal to level 2. Finally, this system attempts to quantify the amount and quality of host bone contact to the implant. Grade I reconstructions represent complete contact between the prosthesis and host bone. Grade II reconstruction has some loss of host-prosthesis contact, but the implant is stable and only morcellized bone graft is required. Grade III loss reveals extensive host-prosthesis contact, requiring structural grafts to stabilize the prosthesis.

PAPROSKY CLASSIFICATION SYSTEM

This system evaluates the femoral diaphysis for its ability to support an uncemented, fully porous-coated prosthesis[10] (Fig. 3). This classification system is less detailed in its description of the bony defect present than the AAOS system, but it is more useful in decision making if an uncemented femoral revision is to be performed. The type I defects are minimal and usually are secondary to an Austin Moore prosthesis or resurfacing procedures. The diaphysis and metaphysis are intact, and there is partial loss of the calcar and anteroposterior (AP) bone stock. Type II bone defects are isolated to the metaphysis with a normal diaphysis. The calcar is completely deficient, and there is major AP bone loss. Type IIIA defects involve the metaphysis and the junction with the diaphysis; however, fixation with a fully porous-coated stem can be achieved proximal to or at the isthmus of the femur. Type IIIB defects extend slightly further than type IIIA; however, reliable fixation can be achieved just past the isthmus of the femur. Finally, type IV defects are extensive with metaphyseal and diaphyseal bone loss and a widened canal that cannot provide adequate fixation to a long stem.

Using this classification system, a preoperative surgical algorithm has been developed by Paprosky. Type I defects are treated as a primary arthroplasty. Type II defects are less likely to lend themselves to cemented or proximally porous-coated stems; a fully coated stem is preferred. Type IIIA defects are treated with a fully coated bowed stem or, less commonly, a straight stem. Type IIIB defects are treated with a fully coated bowed stem or impaction grafting. Type IV femurs are treated with impaction grafting or allograft prosthetic composite (APC). The type IIIB defect is the most difficult to evaluate and requires intraoperative evaluation of the ability of the isthmus to support a fully coated long stem. If it is unable to provide 4 to 6 cm of intimate bone contact, then impaction grafting or an APC will be required as in the type IV femur. If during preoperative templating it appears questionable that the femoral isthmus can support a long, fully porous-coated stem, then the surgeon must treat this case as a type IIIB or type IV femur and be prepared for impaction grafting or the use of an APC.

SURGICAL OPTIONS

The goal of revision surgery is to attempt to reestablish the normal biomechanics of the hip in order to maximize the patient's function. The need for preoperative planning in revision hip surgery cannot be overemphasized. Revision hip surgery is one of the most technical and equipment-intensive types of orthopaedic surgery and is demanding on both the surgeon and the institution. Preparation is the key to a successful outcome, and this begins with a clear understanding of why the hip is being revised and how the revision will be done. The major problem in revision surgery is bone loss that occurs secondary to osteolysis and mechanical factors related to loose components. The remaining bone is often sclerotic and fragile in comparison to bone in a primary arthroplasty.

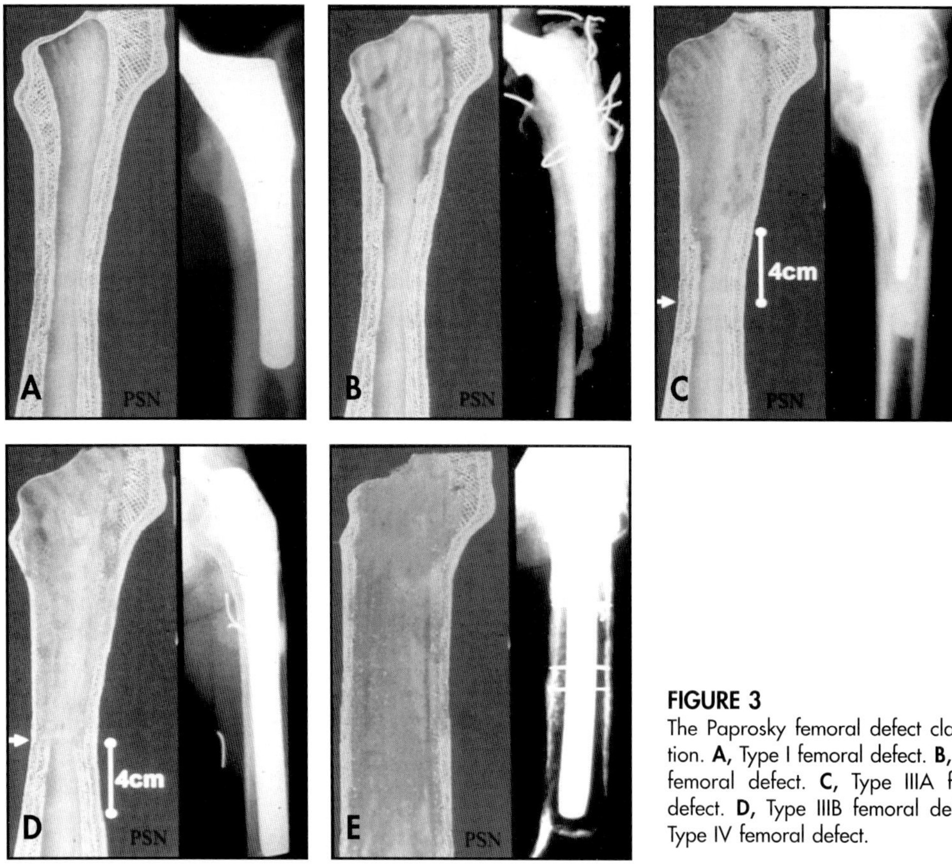

FIGURE 3
The Paprosky femoral defect classification. **A,** Type I femoral defect. **B,** Type II femoral defect. **C,** Type IIIA femoral defect. **D,** Type IIIB femoral defect. **E,** Type IV femoral defect.

Sclerotic bone adversely affects the bond that can be formed between cement and bone because of the lack of interdigitation normally available with a fresh cancellous bed. Bench testing has shown that the shear strength of the bone-cement interface is reduced by 79% in the revision setting.[11] In addition, the revision femur frequently has metaphyseal and diaphyseal defects that preclude achieving a solid cement mantle.

Templating of the femur begins by assessing the bone defect present. The degree and location of bone defects will determine which surgical option and component type will be used. The goal of this surgery is to achieve rotational and axial stability of the femoral construct. Femoral offset should be assessed and restored because it is an important contributor to hip stability. The surgeon should position the component so that the center of the head will be placed to make up any limb-length discrepancy while recreating as normal a center of rotation as possible. It also is important to look for potential conflicts of the prosthesis proximally and on the lateral radiograph. If a stem longer than 7 in is to be used, a conflict with the anterior cortex may exist in the lateral plane, and a curved stem will be needed.

Traditionally, there have been two principal methods of performing revision femoral surgery: cemented and uncemented. Recently, there has been increased interest in rebuilding femoral bone stock through the use of impaction allografting, allograft prosthetic composites, and structural grafting. The Girdlestone technique has been reserved for more severe deficiencies that are not amenable to other reconstruction techniques.

TABLE 1

RESULTS OF CEMENTED FEMORAL REVISION

Authors	Mean Follow-up, Years	Number of Hips	Good/ Excellent Results, %	Re-revision Rate, %	Radiographic Evidence of Femoral Loosening, %
Hunter et al[26]	0.5*	140	24	32% infection rate with 22% resection arth	— —
Amstutz et al[13]	2.1 (mean)	66		9.0	29.0
Pellicci et al[22]	3.4 (mean)	110	60	5.4	13.6
Huo and Salvati[15]	4.1 (mean)	113	83	3.0	16.0
Kavanagh et al[16]	4.5 (mean)	166	52	6.0	44.0
Kilgus et al[18]	5.1 (mean)	92	—	9.0†	—
Mohler et al[20]	5.5 (mean)	96	—	7.0	13.0
Raut et al[23]	7.3 (mean)	39	—	—	5.1
Raut et al[24]	7.5 (mean)	399	—	5.0	7.8
Iorio et al[12]	7.7 (mean)	107	—	3.8	16.0
Pellicci et al[22]	8.1 (mean)	99	63	12.0	29.0
Marti et al[19]	8.9 (mean)	60	—	5.0	32.0
Stromberg et al[27]	10.0 (mean)	51	—	41.0	59.0
Kavanagh et al[17]	10.0 (mean)	210	—	30.0	—
Garcia-Cimbrelo et al[14]	11.5 (mean)	155	—	12% at 10 yr 29% at 10 yr	16% at 16 yr 38% at 16 yr
Callaghan et al[28]	3.6 (mean)	139	66	4.3	12.0
Collis[29]§	4.6 (mean)	110	93	3.6	5.0
Ballard et al[30]§*	5.0 (mean)	27	—	0.0	0.0
Rubash and Harris[31]§*	6.2 (mean)	43	72	4.0	11.0
Weber et al[32]§*	6.2 (mean)	139	—	2.1	8.3
Izquierdo and Northmore-Ball[33]§*	6.5 (mean)	139	—	2.2	4.4
Stromberg and Herberts[25]§*	7.0 (mean)	57	—	7.0	21.0
Pierson and Harris[34]§*	8.5 (mean)	29	86	6.9	14.0
Estok and Harris[35]§*	11.7 (mean)	38	58	10.5	21.0†
Katz et al[36]§*	11.9 (mean)	50	—	9.5	26.0†
Mulroy and Harris[37]§*	15.1 (mean)	35	—	20.0	26.0†

*Minimum follow-up, years
†Combined revision plus loosening rate
§A second-generation cementing technique was used

CEMENTED FEMORAL REVISIONS

As mentioned earlier, a femur with little bone loss in both the metaphyseal and diaphyseal regions (type I Paprosky femur) is amenable to cemented or uncemented revision techniques. Such a choice is available because microinterlock with the cancellous content can occur. More substantial bone loss is dealt with using uncemented implants. Dohmae and associates[11] demonstrated that femurs that had loss of cancellous bone stock had 79% loss of the cement-bone interface shear strength when compared with type I femurs.

Such cautious advice regarding cemented femoral revisions is also based on the cemented revision results that have been published. Most early revisions were performed with cement using first-generation techniques (no pressurization or use of a distal plug) but these had unacceptably high re-revision rates.[12–25] The results are summarized in Table 1.[12–20,22–37] As indicated, the femoral loosening rate was as high as 59%, and the re-revision rate was as high as 41%.[27] Results using such techniques are not easily comparable given the variability in the classification of the preoperative bone defects and the use of a variety of implants including some with sharp corners and narrow medial borders. Of further concern, Hunter and associates[26] reported on a very high failure rate resulting from a high infection rate of 32%, which resulted in a 22% resection arthroplasty rate (Fig. 3).

More recent studies using second generation cementing techniques have demonstrated much better results (Table 1). The only exception is the result from multicenter reports obtained from the Swedish Hip Registry (re-revision rate of 7% and femoral loosening of 21%).[25] The longest-term results are from Mulroy and Harris.[37] At 15 years average follow-up, the femoral loosening rate was 26% while the re-revision rate was 20%. The authors found that the re-revision group was significantly younger at the time of index revision. These results demonstrate a clear improvement in femoral loosening rates with second-generation versus first-generation cementing techniques.

TECHNICAL CONSIDERATIONS

In considering the basic rules surrounding cemented femoral revisions, the major difference in performing a cemented revision as compared to a cemented primary arthroplasty is in the preparation of the femoral canal. The primary setting will have a healthy cancellous bed proximally and good diaphyseal bone distally. In the revision setting, this will not be the case, and the femur will have to be prepared far more thoroughly than in the primary situation. Meticulous removal of all previous cement and pseudomembrane is required. All sclerotic areas of bone and neocortex should be burred down to "fresh" bleeding bone or cancellous bone, being careful to avoid perforation. Pressurization of cement into a plugged canal improves the cement-bone interdigitation. Revision arthroplasties may require more cement than a primary arthroplasty, and two vacuum mixers may be required. The surgeon should then proceed with cementing of the component as in the primary setting (using at least second-generation techniques). This includes at least a 2-mm uniform cement mantle and a 1- to 2-cm cement extension distal to the tip of the stem. The surgeon also should be careful to avoid varus positioning of the stem. There are no data proving that use of third-generation cementing techniques (diminution of cement porosity) clearly improves cemented revision longevity.

UNCEMENTED FEMORAL REVISIONS

The use of uncemented stems in revision arthroplasty has become very prevalent because of the poor results associated with the use of cemented stems. This is particularly true when considering reports of higher failure rates associated with use of long cemented stems, reflecting the poor quality bone stock that was being treated. As mentioned earlier, successful use of cemented stems in the revision setting depends on the presence of adequate metaphyseal and diaphyseal bone in order to obtain good mechanical interlock with host bone.

Uncemented components can be either proximally or fully porous coated. Uncemented components require adequate living bone stock to be in intimate contact with the prosthesis in a mechanically stable setting so that bone ingrowth can occur. The implant must be rotationally and axially stable at the time of implantation to maximize the opportunity for biologic ingrowth. Results of animal studies suggest that bone ingrowth can occur if motion at the bone-implant interface is less than 40 μm; otherwise fibrous ingrowth occurs. There are alternative uncemented implants available, including grit blasted and hydroxyapatite coated stems. Unfortunately, data on their use in the revision setting have not been published.

PROXIMALLY POROUS-COATED IMPLANTS

Proximally porous-coated components aim for fixation in the metaphysis of the femur, which is the area of the femur most commonly damaged secondary to the primary arthroplasty. The metaphysis of the femur also shows the greatest amount of anatomic variability from patient to patient, making it more difficult to achieve stable fixation with intimate bone contact. The distal portion of a proximally coated stem is smooth and cylindrical, with the occasional use of shallow flutes. This design does not offer the torsional stabilty offered with deep cutting flutes or with a slotted flute design. The use of straight stems also does not address the natural anatomic bow of the femur in the AP plane. Thus, bridging of bony defects with a long proximally coated implant will provide limited stability distally.

The use of proximally coated devices in revision surgery has not been successful, with failure rates being as high as 52% and the longest follow-up period being 6.5 years[38] (Table 2). Berry and associates'[39] study was of particular interest given the large number of patients and the comparison of six different proximally coated stem designs. Their 16.5% re-revision rate at a 4.7-year mean follow-up is quite sobering. Failure rates with modular proximal fixation devices such as the S-Rom (Johnson & Johnson, Stanford, CT) have been slightly lower because these implants can closely match the metaphyseal geometry. In addition, this titanium stem theoretically reduces the possibility of stress shielding, and the distal slot provides some torsional stability while reducing the risk of femoral fracture. However, a mechanical loosening rate of 10% at 3 years has been reported.[40]

Devices relying on proximal fixation require good fit and fill of the metaphysis. In the revision setting this area is often sclerotic and fragile, and the dimensions have been enlarged. A proximally porous-coated device can be used if the metaphysis has sufficient bone integrity to allow for rotational and axial stability and if an implant of the correct size can be inserted. With proximal bone destruction, the metaphysial portion of the implant will need to be larger than in a primary arthroplasty. The diaphysis, in contrast, may be undamaged and, as the implant gets larger, it will need to be expanded so that the proximal portion of the implant achieves stability. The ideal would be to achieve both proximal and distal stability; however, proximal stability is crucial for this type of implant.

Before beginning surgery, the ability of the proximal femur to support a proximally porous-coated device must be assessed carefully. The integrity of the proximal femur is maintained by not damaging the greater trochanter or not using an extended trochanteric osteotomy. The surgeon should remove any areas of sclerotic bone that may misdirect reamers or broaches. The greater trochanter may interfere with broaches; therefore, any impinging areas must be carefully removed prior to broaching. The surgeon should use reamers to assess the diaphyseal size, then insert a broach that matches the diaphyseal size and assess this for proximal stability. If the implant is unstable, the surgeon should change the version of the implant or go up to the next implant size, keeping in mind that he or she is now enlarging the diaphysis to achieve proximal fixation. If it appears that going up one or two sizes will achieve proximal fixation, then it may be worthwhile considering this option. However, if an excess amount of diaphysis is being destroyed, it would be better to switch to a fully porous-coated device.

FULLY POROUS-COATED IMPLANTS

Fully porous-coated femoral components obtain their fixation in the diaphysis of the femur and bypass the proximal femur, thus the term bypass fixation is sometimes used to describe this technique. The diaphysis of the femur is able to support a prosthesis in most cases because it usually is affected less by bone defects than is the metaphysis. The diaphysis is also easier to fill with a component because it is a cylinder, and the anatomic variability is greatly reduced. Revisions using this technique have had results approaching those of primary hip arthroplasty with failure rates from 3% to 7% and mean follow-up time up to 13.2 years[41–44] (Table 2).[4,39–41,43–61] Paprosky and associates[44] have reported on a minimum 10 years' clinical and radiographic follow-up of 170 patients with extensively coated cementless revision femoral components. With a range in follow-up of 10 to 16 years and a mean of 13.2 years, a survivorship of over 95% was noted. Clinically, the average Postel-D'Aubigne pain and walking score improved from a preoperative score of 5.4 to 10.8 postoperatively. Of the hips, 82% showed radiographic evidence of a bone-ingrown prosthesis and 13.9% had evidence of stable fibrous fixation. Four percent of the stems were radiographically unstable. Six stems were revised to larger extensively coated stems, and one stem is painful and unstable and has yet to be revised. The overall mechanical failure rate is 4.1% (Fig. 4).

Failures with bypass fixation occur when the canal fill is less than 90% and when less than 4 to 6 cm of diaphysis supports the prosthesis.[62] If these two conditions are met, the success rate is comparable to that of primary arthroplasty. There are two principal disadvantages with this technique; stress shielding and the difficulty of removing a bone-ingrown fully coated stem. Currently, technology limits us to cobalt-chromium (CoCr) for use in extensively porous-coated stems. It has been shown that the stiffer CoCr stems greater than 13.5 mm in diameter are associated with higher degrees of stress shielding. Given that revisions often require the use of larger diameter stems, this is a true concern. Clinically, this has not been an issue that has required re-operation or change in treatment plan. However, should these stems require revision, the challenge will be more daunting given the loss in bone stock proximally and the technical problems associated with removal of fully ingrown stems distally. The availability of titanium devices with extensive textured coating for use in the revision setting may result in lower stress shielding rates. Unfortunately, no long-term results currently are available for these titanium implants.

As mentioned earlier, the goal with bypass fixation is to achieve axial and rotational stability. This can be achieved if at least 4 cm of undisrupted diaphysis is available to support the prosthesis and if greater than 90% canal fill can be achieved.

The surgeon must completely remove all cement, neocortex, and any possible sources of impingement. Reaming must be performed in neutral alignment, and any overhanging trochanter or proximal source of impingement must be removed. In femurs that have remodeled in varus this may not be possible without performing an extended trochanteric osteotomy. Failure to achieve neutral alignment will lead to component malposition or femoral fracture. Thus, the surgeon should perform an extended trochanteric osteotomy if neutral reaming cannot be achieved or if distal observation is required for implant and cement removal.

The length of reaming depends on the stem chosen during the preoperative planning. The surgeon should ream only the area required for fixation and no further. Most reamers have length markers built into them. Fixed reamers are used with straight stems and flexible reamers with curved stems. The femur has an apex anterior bow with the apex approximately 7 in below the lesser trochanter. Therefore, any straight stem longer than 7 in may impinge or perforate the anterior cortex of the femur. Long stems that are curved avoid this potential conflict and have a far lower incidence of anterior cortical perforation than do long straight stems. Reaming is performed sequentially until adequate cortical contact is obtained, keeping in mind the size templated. The surgeon should plan on under-reaming by 0.5 mm. A good test of whether the right size has been chosen is to use a reamer on a T-handle and manually try to turn the reamer

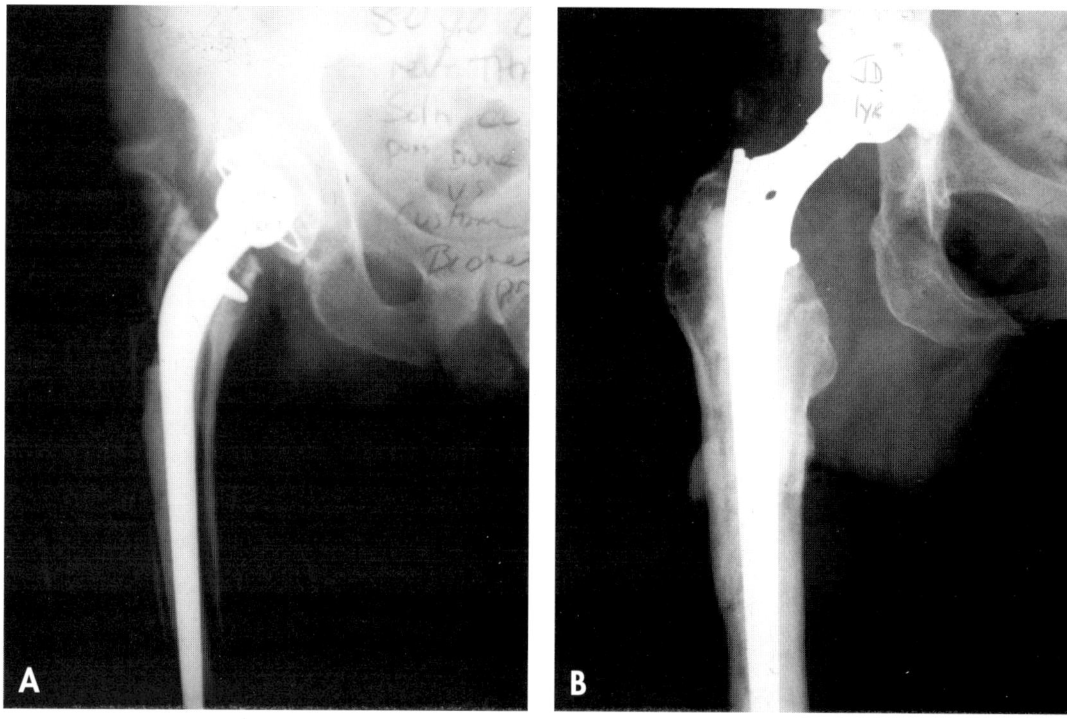

FIGURE 4
Impaction grafting. **A,** Loose cemented femoral component with ectatic femoral canal with diameter greater than 20 mm. **B,** Postoperative impaction grafting with calcar prosthesis.

while it is partially inserted down the canal. If a moderate femoral torque can be achieved using this technique, then the appropriate size has been chosen. For example, if the surgeon has reamed to 16.0 mm with plans to insert a 16.5-mm component, a 16.5-mm reamer on a T-handle is used to test for rotational stability. If rotational stability is not achieved, continue reaming up to the next size.

Before reaming up to the final size, it is important to keep in mind the need to perform trials. In most systems the trial broaches are smaller distally than is the planned stem. For example, a 16.5-mm broach will only be 15.0 mm distally in the Solution system (DePuy, Warsaw, IN). If reaming is performed to 16.0 mm with the intention to implant a 16.5-mm stem, the 16.5-mm broach will not be stable because the distal portion of the broach is only 15.0 mm. Therefore, the surgeon planning on a 16.5-mm stem should ream up to 15.0 mm and perform a trial with the broach before reaming up to 16.0 mm. This size differential will be different for various systems, and the surgeon should keep this in mind because trial reductions with stable broaches are crucial to achieving stability, appropriate component position, and limb lengths.

If an osteotomy has been performed to decrease the chance of fracturing the diaphysis, the surgeon should pass and tighten a cable distal to the osteotomy site before impacting the stem into position. Occasionally, underreaming by 0.5 mm will not be possible, and line to line reaming will be necessary to avoid fracture.

A useful tip is to take the actual prosthesis and use a caliper or a hole gauge to test its actual diameter, and to do the same for the final reamer so that the true size differential between reamer and component is known. Because of manufacturing tolerances and sharpening of the reamers, the size differential may differ significantly from the stated differential.

TABLE 2

RESULTS OF CEMENTLESS FEMORAL REVISION

Authors	Component	Number of Hips	Mean Follow-up, Years	Results
Hedley et al[46]*	PCA	61	1†	9.5% femoral loosening
Harris et al[47]*	Harris-Galante	23	2†	4% femoral loosening
Gustilo and Pasternak[48]*	BIAS	57	2.8	4% femoral revision
Malkani et al[49]	Omnifit	69	3.0	9% re-revision rate
Chandler et al[40]*	S-ROM	52	3.0	4% re-revision rate, 10% mechanical loosening rate
Smith et al[50]*	S-ROM	66	3.4	0% re-revision rate, 7.6% mechanical loosening rate
Cameron[51]*	S-ROM	91	3.5	0% re-revision rate, 2.2% mechanical loosening rate
Meding et al[52]*	PCA and BiMetric	32	3.6	0% re-revision rate, 18% mechanical loosening rate
Trousdale and Morrey[53]*	BIAS	96	4.2	10% re-revision rate 37% subsidence (>2 mm)
Rivero et al[54]*	BIAS	48	4.2	4% re-revision rate 31% subsidence (•4 mm)
Head et al[45]*	Proximal coated/ calcar repl. with struts	174	3 to 9§	3.4 % re-revision rate
Hussamy and Lachiewicz[55]*	BIAS	41	4.5	0% re-revision rate, 32% subsidence (mean, 8 mm)
Mulliken et al[56]*	Mallory-Head	52	4.6	10% re-revision rate 23% mechanical loosening rate
Berry et al[39]*	Proximal porous coating (6 implants)	375	4.7	16.8% re-revision rate for aseptic femoral loosening or osteolysis
Buoncristiani et al[57]*	APR	66	4.7	4.5% re-revision rate
Dorr et al[4]*	APR (collarless)	100	—	50% re-revision rate, 50% subsidence
	APR (collared)	75	—	< 1% re-revision rate, 0% subsidence
McCarthy et al[58]*	S-ROM	133	5	1.5% re-revision rate, 4% subsidence
Woolson et al[38]*	HGP	28	5.5	20% re-revision rate 52% mechanical loosening rate
Peters et al[59]*	BIAS	49	5.5	96% survival rate (6 y)
Jones and Hungerford[60]*	PCA	91	6.5	10% re-revision rate
Engh et al[41]	AML	127	4	4% femoral loosening
Moreland and Bernstein[79]	AML	175	5	2.5% re-revision rate, 2.9% mechanical loosening rate
Lawrence et al[61]	AML	174	8.4	5.7% re-revision, 90.6% survival rate (10 y)
Paprosky et al[44]	Solution	170	13.2	4.1% re-revision rate

*Proximal porous-coated
†Minimum follow-up, years
§Range of follow-up, years
¶Extensively porous-coated

Once the surgeon is satisfied with the size differential, he or she should begin inserting the component by hand, rotating it back and forth to advance it. If more than 5 cm remains proud, it will be necessary to ream line to line. After the component has been advanced as far as possible by hand, the surgeon should begin hitting it with the hammer. At this point, it is crucial to maintain the appropriate anteversion as determined by the trial reduction. Once the prosthesis engages distally in the zone that was underreamed it will be very difficult to change the version.

IMPACTION ALLOGRAFTING

Recently cemented revisions have been performed with the use of impaction grafting, a procedure in which morcellized cancellous bone graft is packed into the canal before cementing a stem. Some consider the use of a polished, collarless, double-tapered stem with a distal centralizer to be crucial for success. The latter allows for subsidence of the implant within the cement mantle, resulting in a radial compression that further impacts the bone graft into the surrounding bone. This technique claims to restore femoral bone stock and can be used with extensive femoral defects. This restoration of femoral bone stock is of particular importance in younger patients who may require future revisions. To date there has been some initial radiographic and histologic evidence of remodeling of the impacted allograft bone. Histologic evidence confirms that there are three zones of bone remodeling, including an outer regenerated cortex, an intermediate region of mixed osteoid and bone cement, and an inner necrotic bone-cement region.[63] Of some concern are reports of early excessive subsidence. In one report, all implants migrated from 0.4 mm to 4.9 mm in the first year.[64] In another study, there was evidence of subsidence in 38% of the cases (average of 10.1 mm).[65] Elting and associates[66] also reviewed 56 individuals at 2 to 5 years; the Harris Hip Score average was 90 points, with > 80% reporting no pain. On radiograph, 48% of the stems showed an average of 2.8 mm of subsidence in the polymethylmethacrylate mantle, but only 7% of the cement graft composites had subsided in the cortical tube. Despite the subsidence, the overall results of this technique are promising.

Early results of impaction grafting have been promising with a re-revision rate ranging from 0% to 6.0% and the femoral loosening rate up to 11.4%[65–69] (Table 3). However, these results have yet to be reproduced at multiple centers, and the longest follow-up available is a 5.5-year mean with a 1.4% re-revision rate and a femoral loosening rate of 5.4%.[69] Recent reports have described a possible concern regarding inadequate cement mantles produced by this technique resulting in some early failures.[70,71] The latter is a technical issue that may be a concern in centers that do not perform this technique on a regular basis. At present, our major indication for this technique is a wide femoral isthmus incapable of providing rotational stability with a fully porous-coated stem (Paprosky type IV) (See Fig. 4).

Impaction grafting uses morcellized cancellous graft to create a neomedullary canal into which a component can be cemented. In creating a new canal, bone graft will be impacted into the femur quite forcefully. The integrity of the femur must be restored so that the femur will tolerate this.

The surgeon must completely expose the proximal femur and clear it of all pseudomembrane, examine the femur for both cavitary and segmental defects, and repair segmental defects to convert them to contained defects using either mesh or strut grafts that are held in place with cerclage wires. If the femur is fragile, it should be cerclage wired prophylactically with multiple cables before impacting bone graft because graft impaction can generate significant hoop stresses. A guide wire is passed through the center of a thick distal medullary plug seated at least 2 cm distal to any lytic lesion. It is imperative that the plug is solidly in place and that the guide wire is neutrally aligned. If necessary, a radiograph should be obtained at this point to ensure the alignment is correct. The bone packing and trial insertion are done with a cannulated system; therefore, the guide wire will dictate the position of the stem. Passing a Kirschner wire transversely through the femur just distal to the plug can prevent distal plug migration. Morcellized

TABLE 3

RESULTS OF CEMENTING WITH IMPACTION GRAFTING

Authors	Component	Number of Hips	Mean Follow-up, Years	Re-revision Rate, %	Radiographic Evidence of Femoral Loosening
Gie et al[67]	Exeter	50	(3.8-6.6)*	0.0	—
Meding et al[65]	Exeter	34	2.5	6.0	38% subsidence (average 10.1 mm)
Elting et al[66]	CPT	56	2.6	0.0	—
Sloof et al[68]	Exeter	88	5.0	—	11.4% failure rate
Elting et al[69]	Exeter & CPT	147	5.5	1.4	5.4%

*Range

cancellous chips should be prepared with a 3- to 5-mm diameter; graft that is too small may compromise the fixation. The surgeon should place the graft into the canal and begin impacting it using cannulated tamps (Fig. 5), packing the bone in a distal to proximal fashion. The final cannulated tamp should be one to two sizes larger than the prosthesis to be used. The bone graft should be packed in very tightly because tight packing is believed to be the key to a successful result. In the end, there should be a uniform 5 to 6 mm of bone around the new canal. The guide wire is then removed. The trials are oversized to allow for a cement mantle, and they should be impacted into place to the appropriate depth determined by trial reduction. The bone packing should be tight enough to prevent removal of the trial by hand, and removal should require a disimpaction force. The cement should be mixed in a standard fashion and introduced in a more liquid state than in primary arthroplasty so that it can penetrate into the bone graft. It is pressurized with a proximal seal.

The stem used by the developers of this technique is a highly polished, collarless, double-tapered design. As mentioned earlier, it is intended to subside in the cement mantle with time, thus "engaging" the cement and further pressurizing the allograft bone. Postoperatively the patients are kept on protected weight bearing for 8 to 12 weeks.

APC AND STRUT GRAFTS

The use of an APC is a very complex undertaking and, fortunately, the need for this is not common even at institutions that do a large number of revisions. Structural allografting is necessary whenever the host femur is incapable of providing stable fixation to a revision component. When there are segmental defects that are of limited length and noncircumferential, strut grafts can be used. When considering noncontained defects involving the calcar region of the proximal femur, a structural allograft will be necessary when there are circumferential defects greater than 5 cm in length. Circumferential segmental defects less than 5 cm in length can be treated with calcar-replacing or long-necked components. An APC also should be considered when there is an extremely large intramedullary defect with a thin cortical shell.

Strut grafts are fairly easily applied and held with cerclage wires. They can be used in many situations to span deficient areas of femoral cortex. Overall, they have shown very reliable rates of healing.[72] However, the theory behind loading of the allograft varies significantly. Head and associates[45] reported that 174 patients were treated with revision total hip arthroplasty, performed by a standardized surgical technique, using cortical onlay strut allografts to restore the structural integrity of the femur and a calcar replacement proximally porous-coated femoral prosthesis composed of titanium alloy. The grafts united 98% of the time and showed evi-

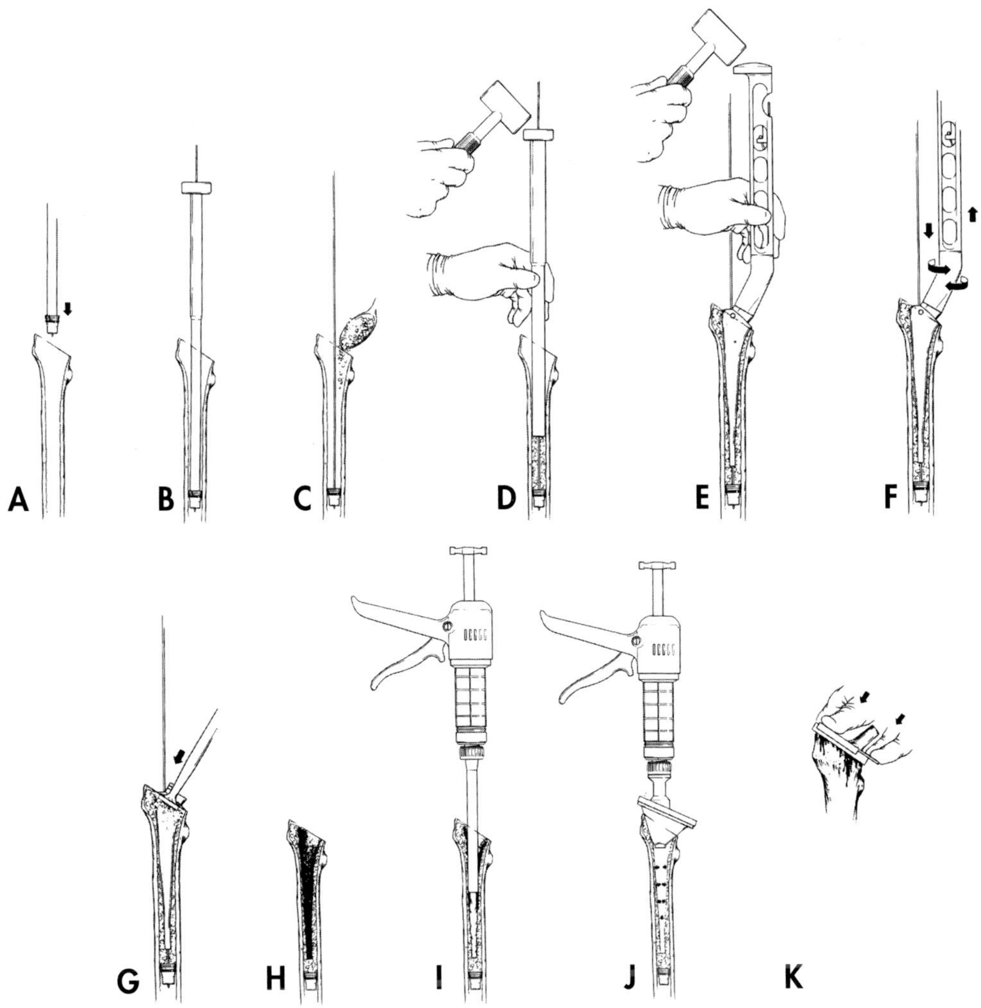

FIGURE 5
The multiple steps of femoral impaction of morcellized allograft bone. The graft is introduced in a retrograde fashion using acannulated impaction sytem. The proximal tamping is completed with a smooth taper tamp. The stem is then cemented into the prepared canal. (Reproduced with permission from Nelissen RGHH, Bauer TW, Weidenhielm LRA, LeGolvan DP, Mikhail WEM: Revision hip arthroplasty with the use of cement and impaction grafting. *J Bone Joint Surg* 1995;77A:412-422.)

dence of revascularization, and in some cases, complete incorporation. They theorize that successful reconstruction of the deficient femur after failed total hip arthroplasty depends on several factors: the revision prosthesis must be stable, the deficient femoral bone stock must be augmented, and load must be transferred to the proximal femur so that the future proximal femoral resorption is minimized. The host femur and allograft will respond physiologically to load bearing, and the graft increases bone quantity and quality. The prosthesis must be supported primarily on host bone; the graft may enhance prosthetic support, but can never be used for primary prosthetic support when using uncemented revision prostheses. Pak and associates[73] also has reported on the use of strut allografts in revision surgery. The technique uses CoCr stems that provide bypass fixation; thus, loading of the graft is not an integral part of the construct. One hundred thirteen cases of cementless femoral revision total hip arthroplasty using either cortical strut or proximal calcar allografts were reviewed for radiographic incorporation at an average of 4.75 years after surgery. All cortical strut grafts were used to supplement the host bone after achieving stable femoral fixation by a tight distal diaphyseal fit. Eighty-seven of the 95 cortical strut grafts showed radiographic evidence of graft incorporation. This points out the controversy that still exists surrounding the amount of loading required when performing a strut allograft procedure.

Bulk proximal allografts are best used with long-stemmed components cemented into the proximal segment and press fit distally into the host. This often requires the use of custom components because the allograft used is often quite narrow although the host femur distally has a large circumference with thin cortices. One of the most important parts of the construct is the junction between allograft and host.[74] This junction may be in the form of a butte joint, step cut, sides sleeve, or with the allograft telescoped into the host distally (Fig. 6). There is no consensus as to which type of junction is the best, but the greater the stability the greater the chance of graft survival. The type of distal cut used depends principally on the rotational stability achieved in the distal femur. Generally, if good rotational stability can be achieved in the distal segment then a butte joint is sufficient. If there is less stability, then a step cut can be used that improves the rotational stability but is technically more difficult to do. The junction also can be supplemented with strut grafts and plates if further stability is required. Whichever junction is used, the surgeon should avoid getting cement into it as much as possible.

Few long-term studies looking specifically at the use of structural femoral allografts are available for review in the literature. Gross and associates[74] have the largest and longest follow-up series of proximal femoral allografts. The success rate in 130 patients with at least 2 years' follow-up was 85%. There were 17 revisions in 16 patients: three revisions for infection, eight for dislocation, five for nonunion, and one for pain. The revision rate is 10.1%. Despite efforts to improve the allograft-host junction healing, a 5.4% nonunion rate was present in this series.

The surgeon should split the remnants of the proximal femur into two, extending this distally to viable and solid bone. The soft-tissue attachments of the proximal femur should be preserved because this bone can be wrapped around the allograft preserving muscular attachments. The surgeon should prepare the allograft to accept the prosthesis that best fits the distal femur without overreaming the allograft. There may be a mismatch between the allograft and host, and a normal distal press fit may not be possible if the allograft is to be preserved. In general, the surgeon should avoid screws into the allograft because this can lead to fracture. It is important that the prosthesis achieve stable fixation in the host distally. If the junction between graft and host is above the isthmus, reliable fixation can be achieved in the isthmus. If the junction is distal to the isthmus or the femur is a Paprosky type IV, isthmus fit will not be possible. In this case, the prosthesis will need to be cemented or fixed with interlocking screws into a custom implant.

POSTOPERATIVE MANAGEMENT

Postoperative management is individualized. The type of postoperative care required depends on the quality of bone noted intraoperatively, the intraoperative bony fixation, and the hip stability. Other factors such as the patient's comorbidity status and motivation are also important variables.

MEDICAL CONSIDERATIONS

Blood management is an important consideration for the orthopaedic surgeon about to perform a revision hip arthroplasty. Because of the increased operative time and extent of surgical exposure, revision surgery is associated with an increased blood loss.[75] The options available to the surgeon include use of the blood bank, autologous blood donation, directed blood donation, a cell-saver

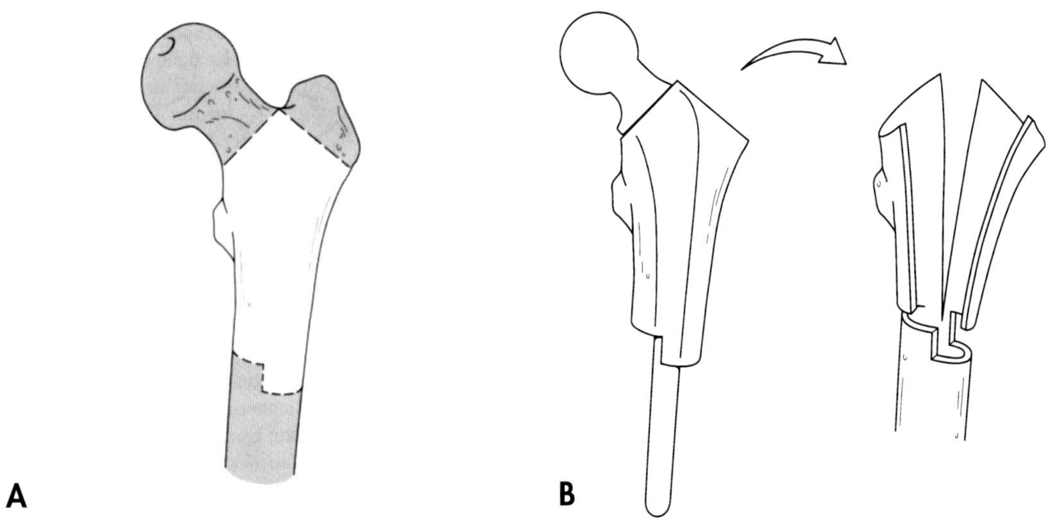

FIGURE 6
A and **B,** Allograft prosthetic composite technique for reconstruction of a severely deficient proximal femur. The allograft bone is shaped and an implant is cemented into the allograft bone. The construct is then impacted into the host bone with fixation being achieved by use of a step cut and cerclage wires. (Reproduced with permission from Hutchison CR, Gross AE: Femoral bone grafting, in Steinberg ME, Garino JP (eds): *Revision Total Hip Arthroplasty.* Philadelphia, PA, Lippincott-Willliams & Wilkins, 1999, pp 263-279.)

system, and reperfusion drains. The use of recombinant erythropoietin is promising and may be cost effective in cases where a great deal of blood loss is anticipated.

Antithrombotic prophylaxis is required to help reduce the high rate of deep venous thrombosis (DVT) associated with total hip arthroplasty. Medical prophylaxis includes warfarin, low-molecular-weight heparin, or aspirin.[76] Mechanical techniques are also used in an adjuvant fashion to prevent thrombosis. These include compressive stockings and pneumatic compressive devices. Despite the multiple regimens available, no single technique has been shown to be clearly better in reducing the DVT rate or, more importantly, the fatal pulmonary embolus rate. Most treatment regimens described are based on 6 weeks of medical management. Given the difficulty in managing warfarin over this time frame, 6 weeks of low-molecular-weight heparin or aspirin treament are gaining in popularity.

Given that all failed total hip arthroplasties run the risk of being infected, surgeons are encouraged to delay administering antibiotics until an adequate intraoperative sample is obtained for culture. Once this is obtained, a broad-spectrum antibiotic can be administered and usually continued for 48 hours.

Postoperative weight bearing after a revision hip arthroplasty is difficult to generalize for all cases and varies from surgeon to surgeon. The most important variables that will help determine the weight bearing status include the quality of bone noted intraoperatively, the intraoperative bony fixation of the implant, and use of any structural graft. In my practice, whenever a porous-coated component is used, weight bearing is restricted to less than 50% body weight for a minimum of 6 weeks. If there are any concerns about the stability of the construct, this period is extended. If structural graft is used on the acetabular reconstruction, the period of restricted weight bearing is extended to a minimum of 12 weeks and may extend for up to 1 year, although this is rare. For patients with cancellous grafting, restricted weight bearing is usually 6 weeks. The use of the extended trochanderic osteotomy does not change our postoperative management.

The dislocation rate after revision total hip arthroplasty is much higher than in the primary setting. Patients are educated about hip precautions, and these are reinforced at each follow-up period. Patients are also placed in a Newport, hip spica-type brace whenever they are out of bed. In those patients who have demonstrated some intraoperative instability, the brace is kept on 24 hours a day for a total of 8 weeks. The restricted range of motion allows for soft-tissue healing and muscle strengthening, thus reducing the chance of dislocation. Under normal circumstances, the Newport brace is worn for a minimum of 6 weeks.

REFERENCES

1. O'Neill DA, Harris WH: Failed total hip replacement: Assessment by plain radiographs, arthrograms, and aspiration of the hip joint. *J Bone Joint Surg* 1984;66A:540-546.
2. Engh CA, Bobyn JD, Glassman AH: Porous-coated hip replacement: The factors governing bone ingrowth, stress shielding, and clinical results. *J Bone Joint Surg* 1987;69B:45-55.
3. Chandler HP, Penenberg BL (eds): *Bone Stock Deficiency in Total Hip Replacement: Classification and Management.* Thorofare, NJ, SLACK, 1989, pp 19-164.
4. Dorr LD, Dierdorf D, Carn RM: Prinicples of cementless total hip revision and use of the APR revision hip. *Tech Orthop* 1987;2:20-33.
5. Engh CA, Glassman AH: Cementless revision of failed total hip replacement. *Orthop Rev* 1990;14 (suppl):23-28.
6. Gross AE, Allan DG, Lavoie GJ, Oakeshott RD: Revision arthroplasty of the proximal femur using allograft bone. *Orthop Clin North Am* 1993;24:705-715.
7. Mallory TH: Preparation of the proximal femur in cementless total hip revision. *Clin Orthop* 1988;235:47-60.
8. Paprosky WG, Bradford MS, Younger TI: Classification of bone defects in failed prostheses. *Chir Organi Mov* 1994;79:285-291.
9. D'Antonio J, McCarthy JC, Bargar WL, et al: Classification of femoral abnormalities in total hip arthroplasty. *Clin Orthop* 1993;296:133-139.
10. Aribindi R, Barba M, Solomon MI, Arp P, Paprosky W: Bypass fixation. *Orthop Clin North Am* 1998;29:319-329.
11. Dohmae Y, Bechtold JE, Sherman RE, Puno RM, Gustilo RB: Reduction in cement-bone interface shear strength between primary and revision arthroplasty. *Clin Orthop* 1988;236:214-220.
12. Iorio R, Eftekhar N, Kobayashi S, Grelsamer RP: Cemented revision of failed total hip arthroplasty: Suvivorship analysis. *Clin Orthop* 1995;316:121-130.
13. Amstutz HC, Ma SM, Jinnah RH, Mai L: Revision of aseptic loose total hip arthroplasties. *Clin Orthop* 1982;170:21-33.
14. Garcia-Cimbrelo E, Munuera L, Diez-Vazquez V: Long-term results of aseptic cemented Charnley revisions. *J Arthroplasty* 1995;10:121-131.
15. Huo MH, Salvati EA: Revision total hip replacement using cement. *Tech Orthop* 1993;7:58-64.
16. Kavanagh BF, Ilstrup DM, Fitzgerald RH Jr: Revision total hip arthroplasty. *J Bone Joint Surg* 1985;67A:517-526.
17. Kavanagh BF, Wallrichs S, Ilstrup D, Berry D, Fitzgerald RH: Ten year follow up of cemented revision total hip replacement. *Orthop Trans* 1993;17:943.
18. Kilgus DJ, Luetzow W, Tipton J, Moreland J, Amstutz H: Factors affecting the outcome of femoral component revision in total hip arthroplasty. *Orthop Trans* 1993;17:966-967.
19. Marti RK, Schuller HM, Besselaar PP, Vanfrank Haasnoot EL: Results of revision of hip arthroplasty with cement: A five- to fourteen-year follow-up study. *J Bone Joint Surg* 1990; 72A: 346-354.
20. Mohler CG, Collis DK: Femoral reconstruction: Cement, in Galante JO, Rosenberg AG, Callaghan JJ (eds): *Total Hip Revision Surgery.* New York, NY, Raven Press, 1995, pp 359-365.
21. Pellicci PM, Wilson PD Jr, Sledge CB, Salvati EA, Ranawat CS, Poss R: Revision total hip arthroplasty. *Clin Orthop* 1982;170:34-41.

22. Pellicci PM, Wilson PD Jr, Sledge CB, et al: Long-term results of revision total hip replacement: A follow-up report. *J Bone Joint Surg* 1985; 67A:513-516.

23. Raut VV, Siney PD, Wroblewski BM: Cemented revision Charnley low-friction arthroplasty in patients with rheumatoid arthritis. *J Bone Joint Surg* 1994;76B:909-911.

24. Raut VV, Siney PD, Wroblewski BM: Outcome of revision for mechanical stem failure using the cemented Charnley's stem: A study of 399 cases. *J Arthroplasty* 1996;11:405-410.

25. Stromberg CN, Herberts P: Cemented revision total hip arthroplasties in patients younger than 55 years old: A multicenter evaluation of second-generation cementing technique. *J Arthroplasty* 1996;11:489-499.

26. Hunter GA, Welsh RP, Cameron HU, Bailey WH: The results of revision of total hip arthroplasty. *J Bone Joint Surg* 1979;61B:419-421.

27. Stromberg CN, Herberts P: A multicenter 10-year study of cemented revision total hip arthroplasty in patients younger than 55 years old: A follow-up report. *J Arthroplasty* 1994;9:595-601.

28. Callaghan JJ, Salvati EA, Pellicci PM, Wilson PD Jr, Ranawat CS: Results of revision for mechanical failure after cemented total hip replacement, 1979 to 1982: A two- to five-year follow-up. *J Bone Joint Surg* 1985;67A:1074-1085.

29. Collis DK: The value of maintaining outcomes in an individual practice for 25 years. *Clin Orthop* 1997;344:69-80.

30. Ballard WT, Callaghan JJ, Johnston RC: Revision of total hip arthroplasty in octogenarians. *J Bone Joint Surg* 1995;77A:585-589.

31. Rubash HE, Harris WH: Revision of nonseptic, loose, cemented femoral components using modern cementing techniques. *J Arthroplasty* 1988;3:241-248.

32. Weber KL, Callaghan JJ, Goetz DD, Johnston RC: Revision of a failed cemented total hip prosthesis with insertion of an acetabular component without cement and a femoral component with cement: A five- to eight-year follow-up study. *J Bone Joint Surg* 1996;78A:982-994.

33. Izquierdo RJ, Northmore-Ball MD: Long-term results of revision hip arthroplasty: Survival analysis with special reference to the femoral component. *J Bone Joint Surg* 1994;76B:34-39.

34. Pierson JL, Harris WH: Cemented revision for femoral osteolysis in cemented arthroplasties: Results in 29 hips after a mean 8.5-year follow-up. *J Bone Joint Surg* 1994;76B:40-44.

35. Estok DM II, Harris WH: Long-term results of cemented femoral revision surgery using second-generation techniques: An average 11.7-year follow-up evaluation. *Clin Orthop* 1994; 299:190-202.

36. Katz RP, Callaghan JJ, Sullivan PM, Johnston RC: Long-term results of revision total hip arthroplasty with improved cementing technique. *J Bone Joint Surg* 1997;79B:322-326.

37. Mulroy WF, Harris WH: Revision total hip arthroplasty with use of so-called second-generation cementing techniques for aseptic loosening of the femoral component: A fifteen-year-average follow-up study. *J Bone Joint Surg* 1996; 78A:325-330.

38. Woolson ST, Delaney TJ: Failure of a proximally porous-coated femoral prosthesis in revision total hip arthroplasty. *J Arthroplasty* 1995;10(suppl): S22-S28.

39. Berry DJ, Harmsen WS, Ilstrup D, Lewallen DG, Cabanela ME: Survivorship of uncemented proximally porous-coated femoral components. *Clin Orthop* 1995;319:168-177.

40. Chandler HP, Ayres DK, Tan RC, Anderson LC, Varma AK: Revision total hip replacement using the S-ROM femoral component. *Clin Orthop* 1995;319:130-140.

41. Engh CA, Glassman AH, Griffin WL, Mayer JG: Results of cementless revision for failed cemented total hip arthroplasty. *Clin Orthop* 1988;235:91-110.

42. Lawrence JM, Engh CA, Macalino GE, Lauro GR: Outcome of revision hip arthroplasty done without cement. *J Bone Joint Surg* 1994;76A: 965-973.

43. Moreland JR, Bernstein ML: Femoral revision hip arthroplasty with uncemented, porous-coated stems. *Clin Orthop* 1995;319:141-150.

44. Paprosky WG, Greidanus NV, Antoniou J: Minimum 10-year-results of extensively porous-coated stems in revision hip arthoplasty. *Clin Orthop* 1999;369:230-242.

45. Head WC, Wagner RA, Emerson RH Jr, Malinin TI: Revision total hip arthroplasty in the deficient femur with a proximal load-bearing prosthesis. *Clin Orthop* 1994;298:119-126.

46. Hedley AK, Gruen TA, Ruoff DP: Revision of failed total hip arthroplasties with uncemented porous-coated anatomic components. *Clin Orthop* 1988;235:75-90.

47. Harris WH, Krushell RJ, Galante JO: Results of cementless revisions of total hip arthroplasties using the Harris-Galante prosthesis. *Clin Orthop* 1988;235:120-126.

48. Gustilo RB, Pasternak HS: Revision total hip arthroplasty with titanium ingrowth prosthesis and bone grafting for failed cemented femoral component loosening. *Clin Orthop* 1988; 235:111-119.

49. Malkani AL, Lewallen DG, Cabanela ME, Wallrichs SL: Femoral component revision using an uncemented, proximally coated, long-stem prosthesis. *J Arthroplasty* 1996;11:411-418.

50. Smith JA, Dunn HK, Manaster BJ: Cementless femoral revision arthroplasty: 2- to 5-year results with a modular titanium alloy stem. *J Arthroplasty* 1997;12:194-201.

51. Cameron HU: The two- to six-year results with a proximally modular noncemented total hip replacement used in hip revisions. *Clin Orthop* 1994;298:47-53.

52. Meding JB, Ritter MA, Keating EM, Faris PM: Clinical and radiographic evaluation of long-stem femoral components following revision total hip arthroplasty. *J Arthroplasty* 1994;9:399-408.

53. Trousdale RT, Morrey BF: Uncemented femoral revision of total hip arthroplasty. *Orthop Trans* 1993;17:964-965.

54. Rivero D, Jacobs JJ, Galante JO, Rosenberg AG: Revision cementless total hip arthroplasty: Two to five year results. *Orthop Trans* 1993;17:171.

55. Hussamy O, Lachiewicz PF: Revision total hip arthroplasty with the BIAS (Biologic Ingrowth Anatomic System) femoral component: Three- to six-year results. *J Bone Joint Surg* 1994; 76A:1137-1148.

56. Mulliken BD, Rorabeck CH, Bourne RB: Uncemented revision total hip arthroplasty: A 4- to-6-year review. *Clin Orthop* 1996;325:156-162.

57. Buoncristiani AM, Dorr LD, Johnson C, Wan Z: Cementless revision of total hip arthroplasty using the anatomic porous replacement revision prosthesis. *J Arthroplasty* 1997;12:403-415.

58. McCarthy JC, Mattingly D, Turner RH, Bierbaum B, Chandler HP, Cameron HU: Revision of the deficient femur with a modular femoral component. *Orthop Trans* 1993;17:966.

59. Peters CL, Rivero DP, Kull LR, Jacobs JJ, Rosenberg AG, Galante JO: Revision total hip arthroplasty without cement: Subsidence of proximally porous-coated femoral components. *J Bone Joint Surg* 1995;77A:1217-1226.

60. Hungerford DS, Jones LC: The rationale of cementless revision of cemented arthroplasty failures. *Clin Orthop* 1988;235:12-24.

61. Lawrence JM, Engh CA, Macalino GE: Revision total hip arthroplasty: Long-term results without cement. *Orthop Clin North Am* 1993;24:635-644.

62. Krishnamurthy AB, MacDonald SJ, Paprosky WG: 5- to 13-year follow-up study on cementless femoral components in revision surgery. *J Arthroplasty* 1997;12:839-847.

63. Ling RS, Timperley AJ, Linder L: Histology of cancellous impaction grafting in the femur: A case report. *J Bone Joint Surg* 1993; 75B: 693-696.

64. Gie GA, Linder L, Ling RSM, Simon JP, Slooff TJ, Timperley AJ: Femoral reconstruction: Cement with graft, in Galante JO, Rosenberg AG, Callaghan JJ (eds): *Total Hip Revision Surgery.* New York, NY, Raven Press, 1995, pp 367-373.

65. Meding JB, Ritter MA, Keating EM, Faris PM: Impaction bone-grafting before insertion of a femoral stem with cement in revision total hip arthroplasty: A minimum two-year follow-up study. *J Bone Joint Surg* 1997;79A:1834-1841.

66. Elting JJ, Mikhail WE, Zicat BA, Hubbell JC, Lane LE, House B: Preliminary report of impaction grafting for exchange femoral arthroplasty. *Clin Orthop* 1995;319:159-167.

67. Gie GA, Linder L, Ling RS, Simon JP, Slooff TJ, Timperley AJ: Impacted cancellous allografts and cement for revision total hip arthroplasty. *J Bone Joint Surg* 1993;75B:14-21.

68. Slooff TJ, Buma P, Schreurs BW, Schimmel JW, Huiskes R, Gardeniers J: Acetabular and femoral reconstruction with impacted graft and cement. *Clin Orthop* 1996;324:108-115.

69. Elting JJ, Raimondo RA, Smallman TV, Hubbell MJ: Abstract: Impaction grafting for femoral revision: 5-year results. Proceedings of the American Academy of Orthopaedic Surgeons 65th Annual Meeting, New Orleans, LA. Rosemont, IL, American Academy of Orthopaedic Surgeons, 1998, p 185.

70. Masterson EL, Masri BA, Duncan CP: The cement mantle in the Exeter impaction allografting technique: A cause for concern. *J Arthroplasty* 1997;12:759-764.

71. Masterson EL, Masri BA, Duncan CP, Rosenberg A, Cabanela M, Gross M: The cement mantle in femoral impaction allografting: A comparison of three systems from four centres. *J Bone Joint Surg* 1997;79B:908-913.

72. Head WC, Malinin TI, Mallory TH, Emerson RH Jr: Onlay cortical allografting for the femur. *Orthop Clin North Am* 1998;29:307-312.

73. Pak JH, Paprosky WG, Jablonsky WS, Lawrence JM: Femoral strut allografts in cementless revision total hip arthroplasty. *Clin Orthop* 1993; 295:172-178.

74. Gross AE, Hutchison CR, Alexeeff M, Mahomed N, Leitch K, Morsi E: Proximal femoral allografts for reconstruction of bone stock in revision arthroplasty of the hip. *Clin Orthop* 1995; 319:151-158.

75. Barrack RL: Economics of revision total hip arthroplasty. *Clin Orthop* 1995;319:209-214.

76. Zimlich RH, Fulbright BM, Friedman RJ: Current status of anticoagulation therapy after total hip and total knee arthroplasty. *J Am Acad Orthop Surg* 1996;4:54-62.

REVISION OF THE INFECTED TOTAL HIP ARTHROPLASTY

JOHN ANTONIOU, MD, PhD

INTRODUCTION

The incidence of deep postoperative infection complicating total hip arthroplasty has diminished from 7% to 10% in the late 1970s to about 1% for primary total hip arthroplasty using modern aseptic surgical techniques (specialized centers have reported an incidence as low as 0.06%).[1,2] Despite this improvement for primary arthroplasty, the rate in revision surgery remains between 2% and 4%. Given the serious nature of this pathology, early diagnosis and appropriate treatment are crucial.

DIAGNOSIS AND EVALUATION

There is no one single diagnostic modality that is a gold standard for deep infection following total hip arthroplasty. The onus is on the surgeon to compile clinical evidence consistent with an underlying infection. The diagnostic tools at the surgeon's disposal include an accurate history, physical examination, laboratory investigations, radiographic evaluation, and intraoperative tests. The laboratory investigations include white blood cell count, erythrocyte sedimentation rate (ESR), and C-reactive protein (CRP). The radiographic evaluation includes plain radiographs, hip joint arthrography and aspiration, and scintigraphic modalities. Finally, the intraoperative tests include aspiration, Gram stain, frozen section, and cultures.

CLASSIFICATION

A detailed history and physical examination must be obtained to accurately assess the possibility of infection and to classify the type of infection being represented. The most widely accepted classification of postoperative hip arthroplasty infection was introduced by Coventry[3] in 1975. The postoperative infections are divided into three stages.

Stage I infection is an acute postoperative infection. This type of infection does not represent a diagnostic problem. The febrile patient presents with a purulent, red, and swollen postoperative wound. The challenge with this type of infection is to determine whether the infection is superficial or deep. The only way to make sure of this determination is a direct inspection of the fascia.

Stage II infection is an indolent, delayed deep infection that occurs 6 months to 2 years after arthroplasty. The patient presents with a painful arthroplasty usually associated with a normal postoperative course. Given that the pain may not be associated with a history of fever, chills, or postoperative wound problems, the surgeon must differentiate stage II infection from other causes of pain such as aseptic loosening. This differentiation can be achieved by using the investigative methods mentioned below.

Stage III infection is a late hematogenous infection occurring 2 or more years after surgery and is usually an easy diagnosis to make. It is important to determine whether the patient underwent a recent surgical intervention, dental procedure, or had a recent infection. The classic presentation is that of a febrile state accompanied by a painful arthroplasty. The diagnostic tests described below usually confirm the suspicion. There have been other classification schemes that have recently been elucidated including that of Schmalzried and associates,[4] which is based on clinical history and laboratory findings, and another by

Tsukayama and associates.[5] With new understanding of organisms and new antibiotic therapies, the classification schemes will evolve. The surgeon must always keep in mind that with evolution must come consensus to maintain uniformity in the way infection is classified and treated.

LABORATORY STUDIES

It is widely accepted that the white blood cell count and differential are of little diagnostic value in the absence of obvious infection. ESR elevation is not very specific, and thus its clinical usefulness is also limited. The use of ESR is most helpful in its negative predictive value (ie, ESR < 30 mm/h is indicative of no infection), which has been reported at 95%.[6] Unfortunately, many factors can cause an elevated ESR, including the first year after arthroplasty, inflammatory arthritis, any infection, and some malignancy. The average ESR sensitivity has been reported at 83% with an accuracy of 80%.[6]

CRP has been described as a very useful acute-phase reactant in the evaluation of infection. Although CRP is susceptible to conditions that cause an increase in acute-phase reactants, it decreases sooner after infection has resolved than does the ESR.[7] The CRP sensitivity (96%) and specificity (92%) are also much higher than those of the ESR.[6] Some have argued that a combined use of these blood tests may increase their accuracy.

RADIOGRAPHIC EVALUATION

Changes noted on plain radiographs such as radiolucent lines or endosteal erosion are not pathognomonic of septic loosening.[8] On the rare occasion, a lacy periosteal new-bone formation may be noted in the infected hip (Fig. 1). Overall, the usefulness of this modality is controversial.

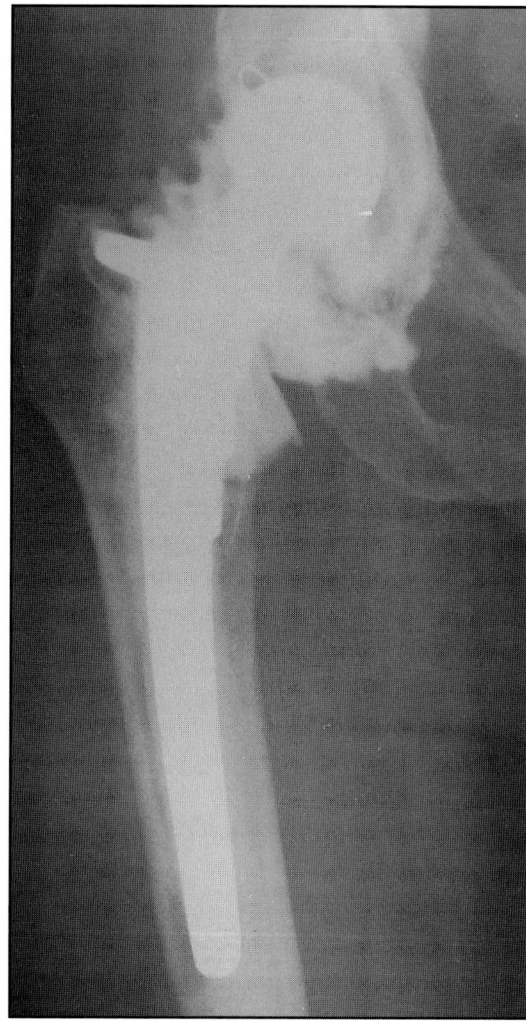

FIGURE 1
A 51-year-old man with an infected total hip arthoplasty demonstrating medial pooling of arthrogram dye in the pseudocapsule. (Reproduced with permission from Fitzgerald RH Jr: Infected total hip arthroplasty: Diagnosis and treatment. *J Am Acad Orthop Surg* 1995;3:249-262.)

Although rarely seen, arthrography can demonstrate pocketing of radiopaque medium in the area of the pseudocapsule, suggesting infection.[8] Thus, hip joint arthrography usually is combined with aspiration to increase its clinical usefulness. Aspiration cannot be used only for the purpose of isolating a potential organism; it also is used for analyzing the white blood cell count and differential, and glucose and protein levels. A white blood cell count of over 25,000/mm^3, a differential blood cell count of over 25% polymorphonuclear leukocytes, and low glucose and protein levels are highly suspicious of underlying infection. The higher the white blood cell count, the higher the likelihood of infection. The sensitivity of preoperative aspirations in clinically suspicious cases has been noted at 86% and the specificity at 94%.[6] Despite the useful clinical data that can be obtained, routine use of this invasive procedure remains controversial. This is especially true when considering the possibility of contamination. Some state that all symptomatic hip failures should undergo an aspiration and arthrography, whereas others argue that their routine use is not cost-effective and should be avoided.[9] Recently, Barrack and Harris[8] reviewed a series of 270 aspirations performed on loosened implants that resulted in a 2% proven infection rate and a 13% false-positive rate. My recommendation is to use aspiration in cases in which infection is clinically suspected but not proven.

SCINTIGRAPHIC EVALUATION

Although much work has been performed attempting to understand the usefulness of scintigraphic evaluation, many contradictory results cloud the issue. Traditional three-phase technetium Tc99m bone scan generally has not proven to be useful for predicting sepsis. It is associated with a high sensitivity but low specificity.[10] Gallium-67 scans also have been disappointing in the diagnosis of infected total hip replacement.

The introduction of indium-111 labeling of autologous white blood cells has proved to be even more sensitive than technetium Tc99m or Gallium-67 in the diagnosis of infected arthroplasty.[11] Unfortunately, even this modality has come under question, and some now argue that a combined bone and indium-111 scan may improve both the sensitivity and specificity in diagnosing infected total joints.[12,13] In addition, this scan is still highly specialized, not universally available, and technician dependent. A new modality of indium-111 labeling immunoglobulin has the potential of having more specific affinity for acute inflammation than labeled white blood cells. In some recent studies, the sensitivity has been quoted at 75% and the specificity at 96%.[14,15] Further studies are required to completely understand the potential usefulness of this new technique.

INTRAOPERATIVE EVALUATION

Intraoperative aspiration has the same potential value as preoperative aspiration. As mentioned previously, a white blood cell count of over 25,000/mm^3, a differential blood cell count of over 25% polymorphonuclear leukocytes, and low glucose and protein levels are suggestive of infection. However, this evaluation alone is not enough to confirm the diagnosis.

Use of Gram stains in the operating room is widespread but has a very questionable usefulness.[16] The false-negative rate has been shown to be unacceptably high. Frozen sections also have been used extensively during revision arthroplasty. Unfortunately, there is variability as to what is considered a positive result; anything from five to ten polymorphonuclear leukocytes per high-power field has been considered to be significant.[6,17-19] Using these criteria, the sensitivity has varied from 80% to 100%, and the specificity has varied from 94% to 99%. Of course, use of this technique is highly dependent on a pathology team that is familiar with what the surgeon is looking for.

Intraoperative cultures have long been considered the gold standard for diagnosing an infected arthroplasty and identifying the causative organism. Given the possibility of sampling error or contamination, some have advocated obtaining at least two samples at the time of surgery. This approach has yielded a sensitivity of 94% and a specificity of 97%.[6]

MICROBIOLOGY OF THE INFECTED TOTAL HIP ARTHROPLASTY

With the advent of highly prevalent antimicrobial therapy, the profile of organisms being isolated from septic hip arthroplasties has been changing. The probable infecting organism to consider depends on the Coventry stage of infection being considered.[3] Stage I infection in the first several postoperative weeks usually is a virulent organism infection resulting from a breach in aseptic conditions during the perioperative period. Stage II infections usually are the result of intraoperative infection with a less virulent organism, usually coagulase negative staphylococci. Stage III infections usually occur over 2 years after surgery and are a result of hematogenous seeding. The type of organism to consider in this situation depends on the source of the bacteremia (ie, streptococcus in the case of dental procedures or enterococci in the case of gastrointestinal procedures). Despite these considerations, the most frequent organisms isolated (> 40% of cases) are gram-positive cocci with *Staphylococcus epidermidis* being twice as common as *S aureus*. Organisms responsible for total hip arthroplasty infection have been developing increased resistance to standard antibiotic therapy. The resistance in the arthroplasty setting has been the result of an indiscriminant use of antibiotics and the creation by the infecting organism of a biofilm layer adjacent to the implant (glycocalyx).[20] The glycocalyx inhibits the penetration of the antimicrobial agent, and it also tends to inactivate the inhibitory or cidal activity of the agent. Given the organism's tendency to produce glycocalyx once a chronic infection has set in, the tendency is for surgeons to remove the implant for adequate treatment of the infection.

TREATMENT

Once the patient has been staged and the appropriate diagnostic modalities have been performed, the surgeon must then decide on the appropriate treatment. There are several treatment options, including debridement, followed by antibiotic therapy, one-stage exchange, two-stage exchange (with or without prostalac spacer), and chronic suppressive antibiotic therapy. The major determinants of treatment include the patient's physical ability to undergo extensive surgical intervention, the patient's immune status, the stage of infection, and the infecting pathogen.

DEBRIDEMENT AND ANTIBIOTIC THERAPY

Traditionally, infected postoperative hematomas (stage I infection)[21] and late hematogenous infections (stage III infections) have been treated with surgical debridement and parenteral antibiotic therapy for 4 to 6 weeks. In the case of a stage I infection, this type of treatment has produced excellent results. Even though many surgeons believe that treating a previously well-functioning hip with a stage III infection in this manner is the treatment of choice,[22-25] there is growing belief that this is not adequate treatment and that the patient will ultimately require removal of the infected implant. It is also believed that the more virulent the infecting organism is, the higher the likelihood that simple debridement will not be enough and that implant removal will be necessary.

Regardless of the method required to diminish the pathogen load, all treatments involve antibiotic therapy. The type and length of antibiotic therapy depend on the type and susceptibility of the organism and the patient's immune status. It is generally believed that a minimum of 4 to 6 weeks of parenteral antibiotic treatment is required to treat infected arthroplasties. Usually, the more virulent the organism, the more aggressive the antimicrobial therapy and the longer the duration of treatment. Depending on the susceptibility of an organism to a well-absorbed oral antibiotic, the treating physician may elect to continue the treatment with oral therapy once the initial 4- to 6-week parenteral treatment is completed. Regardless of the treatment used, close communication with an infectious disease specialist is recommended.

ONE-STAGE REVISION ARTHROPLASTY

Buchholz and Gartmann[26] introduced the concept of one-step exchange arthroplasty. This procedure is based on removing the implant, debriding the affected region, and reimplanting a prosthesis with antibiotic-laden cement. The cement of choice for this procedure, because of its superior elution properties, is Palacos bone cement (Kulzer, Wehrheim, Germany).[27] Different antimicrobial agents have distinct elution properties, with aminoglycosides demonstrating the most prolonged and sustained local antibiotic levels. Despite this variability, antibiotics to be included in the cement should be based on the organism's susceptibility.[8,28,29]

Buchholz and associates'[30] original work reported on successful eradication of infection in

449 of 583 patients. It has subsequently been determined that more virulent bacteria respond less favorably to this treatment. This is especially true in the case of gram-negative bacteria, which are associated with a greater than 50% recurrence rate. Research attempting to identify which organisms would respond to this type of therapy has brought forth the possibility that glycocalyx may be the determining factor. With this in mind, one-stage procedures are now performed in patients with organisms susceptible to an antibiotic and an organism that does not elaborate glycocalyx.

TWO-STAGE EXCHANGE ARTHROPLASTY

This technique remains the treatment of choice among orthopaedic surgeons in North America. McDonald and associates[24] reported that use of this technique resulted in an 85% success rate at 5.5 years. They also demonstrated that the recurrence of infection was reduced if a 3-month interval elapsed between the resection and re-implantation. In the case of more virulent organisms, a 1-year interval was required to produce reasonable results. Determination of whether the infection is eradicated is difficult and requires clinical judgment and serial assessment of CRP and ESR. As mentioned earlier, the use of nuclear studies also can be helpful (Fig. 2).

Adjuvant therapy in the form of implanted polymethylmethacrylate beads loaded with antibiotics has been used to effectively eradicate the remaining organisms. Although it is popular, there is no randomized prospective study clearly proving that this technique is necessary or effective.

Masri and associates[31] introduced a technique aimed at obviating the need for walking with a painful Girdlestone hip. Their concept involves the insertion of a temporary prosthesis coated with antibiotic-impregnated cement. The key to this technique relies on the insertion of the

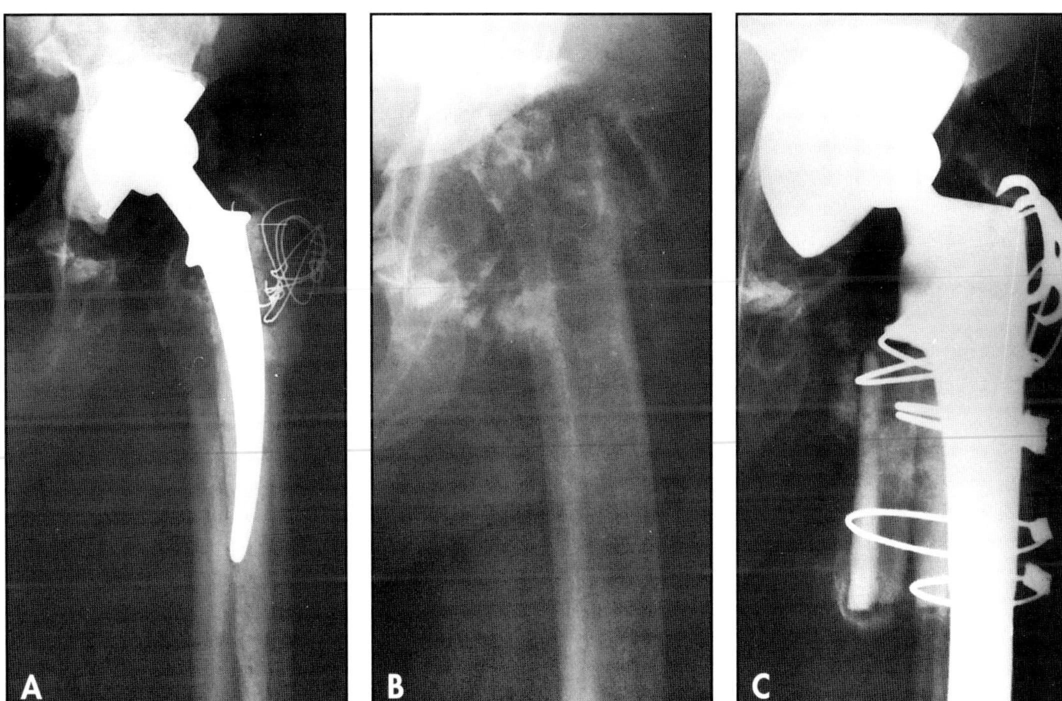

FIGURE 2
A 50-year-old man 10 years after surgery suffered an infected total hip arthroplasty secondary to group D streptococcus and *Staphylococcus epidermidis* organisms. A staged revision arthroplasty was performed with the cementless component being placed at 1 year after resection arthroplasty. (Reproduced with permission from Fitzgerald RH Jr: Infected total hip arthroplasty: Diagnosis and treatment. *J Am Acad Orthop Surg* 1995;3:249-262.)

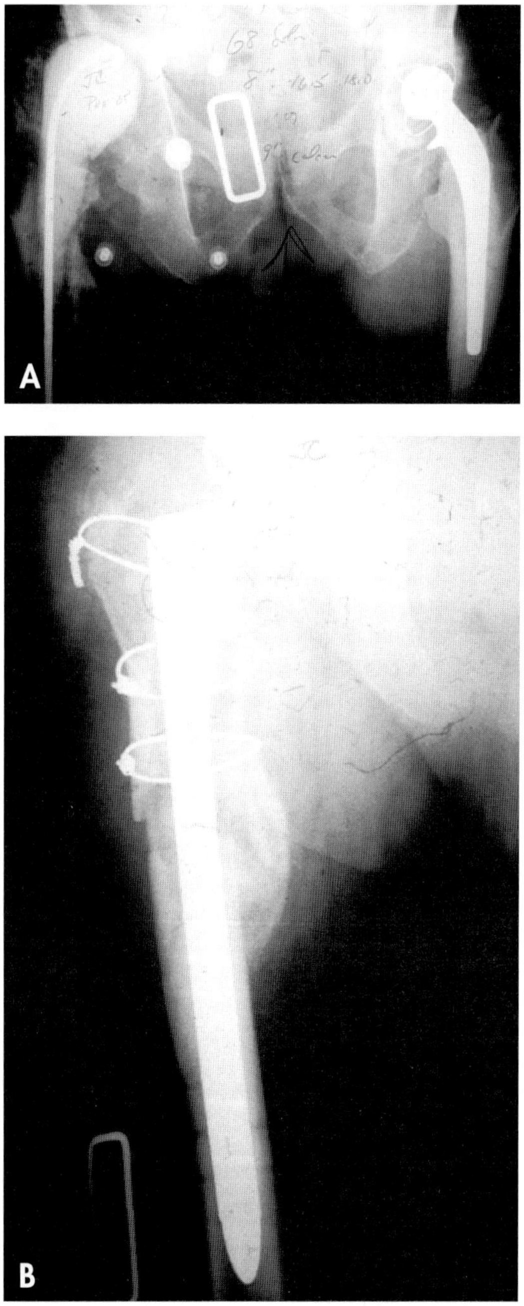

FIGURE 3
A, Prosthetic reconstruction following explanation of infected femoral component. **B,** Reimplantation post removal of prostalic using extensively coated cementless femoral component.

cement-coated implant while the cement has a very doughy consistency. The latter ensures that there will not be a tight seal created at the bone-cement interface. Their reported success rate has been as high as 93% (Fig. 3).

When comparing success of one-stage versus two-stage techniques, the general consensus is that the overall rate of success of delayed reimplantations is greater than that of one-stage procedures. The overall success rate of primary exchanges is approximately 80% if antibiotic-laden cement is used versus 70% if antibiotics are not used. The success rate of two-stage implantation is approximately 90%.[30,32-34] A comparison of the results is given in Table 1.[35-38] Thus, as mentioned earlier, the true indication for a one-stage procedure is a patient with organisms susceptible to an antibiotic and an organism that does not elaborate glycocalyx.

After successful eradication of the organism, reimplantation can be successfully achieved with a cemented implant laden with antibiotics or with a cementless implant using standard revision arthroplasty techniques. There are no prospective randomized studies comparing these techniques.

Permanent resection arthroplasty is considered a procedure of last resort and has been associated with less than perfect clinical function despite its effectiveness in eradicating infections. It is

TABLE 1

RESULTS OF ONE-STAGE VERSUS TWO-STAGE REIMPLANTATION

Authors	Results
Elson[35]	3 times greater failure among primary versus two-stage revisions
Salvati et al[36]	6% versus 10% to 15% recurrence for two-stage versus primary revisions
Garvin et al[37,38]	91% and 82% success when antibiotics were and were not used in two-stage revision versus 82% and 58% success when antibiotics were and were not used in primary revisions

reserved for patients who are immunosuppressed, who cannot medically tolerate a re-implantation procedure, or have other circumstances that put them at risk for re-infection (ie, another source that may lead to hematogenous seeding).

REFERENCES

1. Fitzgerald RH Jr: Total hip arthroplasty sepsis: Prevention and diagnosis. *Orthop Clin North Am* 1992;23:259-264.
2. Lidwell OM, Lowbury EJ, Whyte W, Blowers R, Stanley SJ, Lowe D: Effect of ultraclean air in operating rooms on deep sepsis in the joint after total hip or knee replacement: A randomised study. *Br Med J (Clin Res Ed)* 1982;285:10-14.
3. Coventry MB: Treatment of infections occurring in total hip surgery. *Orthop Clin North Am* 1975; 6:991-1003.
4. Schmalzried TP, Amstutz HC, Au MK, Dorey FJ: Etiology of deep sepsis in total hip arthroplasty: The significance of hematogenous and recurrent infections. *Clin Orthop* 1992;280:200-207.
5. Tsukayama DT, Estrada R, Gustilo RB: Infection after total hip arthroplasty: A study of the treatment of one hundred and six infections. *J Bone Joint Surg* 1996;78A:512-523.
6. Spangehl MJ, Masri BA, O'Connell JX, Duncan CP: Prospective analysis of preoperative and intraoperative investigations for the diagnosis of infection at the sites of two hundred and two revision total hip arthroplasties. *J Bone Joint Surg* 1999;81A:672-683.
7. Shih LY, Wu JJ, Yang DJ: Erythrocyte sedimentation rate and C-reactive protein values in patients with total hip arthroplasty. *Clin Orthop* 1987;225:238-246.
8. Barrack RL, Harris WH: The value of aspiration of the hip joint before revision total hip arthroplasty. *J Bone Joint Surg* 1993;75A:66-76.
9. Lachiewicz PF, Rogers GD, Thomason HC: Aspiration of the hip joint before revision total hip arthroplasty: Clinical and laboratory factors influencing attainment of a positive culture. *J Bone Joint Surg* 1996;78A:749-754.
10. Reing CM, Richin PF, Kenmore PI: Differential bone-scanning in the evaluation of a painful total joint replacement. *J Bone Joint Surg* 1979; 61A:933-936.
11. Pring DJ, Henderson RG, Rivett AG, Krausz T, Coombs RR, Lavender JP: Autologous granulocyte scanning of painful prosthetic joints. *J Bone Joint Surg* 1986;68B:647-652.
12. Johnson JA, Christie MJ, Sandler MP, Parks PF Jr, Homra L, Kaye JJ: Detection of occult infection following total joint arthroplasty using sequential technetium-99m HDP bone scintigraphy and indium-111 WBC imaging. *J Nucl Med* 1988; 29:1347-1353.
13. Palestro CJ, Kim CK, Swyer AJ, Capozzi JD, Solomon RW, Goldsmith SJ: Total-hip arthroplasty: Periprosthetic indium-111-labeled leukocyte activity and complementary technetium-99m-sulfur colloid imaging in suspected infection. *J Nucl Med* 1990;31:1950-1955.
14. Oyen WJ, Claessens RA, van der Meer JW, Corstens FH: Detection of subacute infectious foci with indium-111-labeled autologous leukocytes and indium-111-labeled human nonspecific immunoglobulin G: A prospective comparative study. *J Nucl Med* 1991; 32:1854-1860.
15. Oyen WJ, van Horn JR, Claessens RA, Slooff TJ, van der Meer JW: Diagnosis of bone, joint, and joint prosthesis infections with In-111-labeled nonspecific human immunoglobulin G scintigraphy. *Radiology* 1992;182:195-199.
16. Chimento GF, Finger S, Barrack RL: Gram stain detection of infection during revision arthroplasty. *J Bone Joint Surg* 1996;78B:838-839.
17. Feldman DS, Lonner JH, Desai P, Zuckerman JD: The role of intraoperative frozen sections in revision total joint arthroplasty. *J Bone Joint Surg* 1995;77A:1807-1813.
18. Lonner JH, Desai P, Dicesare PE, Steiner G, Zuckerman JD: The reliability of analysis of intraoperative frozen sections for identifying active infection during revision hip or knee arthroplasty. *J Bone Joint Surg* 1996;78A:1553-1558.
19. Mirra JM, Amstutz HC, Matos M, Gold R: The pathology of the joint tissues and its clinical relevance in prosthesis failure. *Clin Orthop* 1976; 117:221-240.

20. Kloos WE, Bannerman TL: Update on clinical significance of coagulase-negative staphylococci. *Clin Microbiol Rev* 1994;7:117-140.

21. Fitzgerald RH Jr: Diagnosis and management of the infected hip prosthesis. *Orthopedics* 1995; 18:833-835.

22. Charnley J: The future of total hip replacement. *Hip* 1982;198-210.

23. Hunter G, Dandy D: The natural history of the patient with an infected total hip replacement. *J Bone Joint Surg* 1977;59B:293-297.

24. McDonald DJ, Fitzgerald RH Jr, Ilstrup DM: Two-stage reconstruction of a total hip arthroplasty because of infection. *J Bone Joint Surg* 1989; 71A:828-834.

25. Nelson CL, Evarts CM, Andrish J, Marks K: Results of infected total hip replacement arthroplasty. *Clin Orthop* 1980;147:258-261.

26. Buchholz HW, Gartmann HD: Infection prevention and surgical management of deep insidious infection in total endoprosthesis. *Chirurg* 1972;43:446-453.

27. Hoff SF, Fitzgerald RH Jr, Kelly PJ: The depot administration of penicillin G and gentamicin in acrylic bone cement. *J Bone Joint Surg* 1981; 63A:798-804.

28. Hill C, Flamant R, Mazas F, Evrard J: Prophylactic cefazolin versus placebo in total hip replacement: Report of a multicentre double-blind randomised trial. *Lancet* 1981;1:795-796.

29. Mauerhan DR, Nelson CL, Smith DL, et al: Prophylaxis against infection in total joint arthroplasty: One day of cefuroxime compared with three days of cefazolin. *J Bone Joint Surg* 1994; 76A:39-45.

30. Buchholz HW, Elson RA, Engelbrecht E, Lodenkamper H, Rottger J, Siegel A: Management of deep infection of total hip replacement. *J Bone Joint Surg* 1981;63B:342-353.

31. Masri BA, Duncan CP, Beauchamp CP: Long-term elution of antibiotics from bone-cement: An in vivo study using the prosthesis of antibiotic-loaded acrylic cement (PROSTALAC) system. *J Arthroplasty* 1998;13:331-338.

32. Garvin KL, Fitzgerald RH Jr, Salvati EA, et al: Reconstruction of the infected total hip and knee arthroplasty with gentamicin-impregnated Palacos bone cement, in Heckman JD (ed): *Instructional Course Lectures 42.* Rosemont, IL, American Academy of Orthopaedic Surgeons, 1993, pp 293-302.

33. Hope PG, Kristinsson KG, Norman P, Elson RA: Deep infection of cemented total hip arthroplasties caused by coagulase-negative staphylococci. *J Bone Joint Surg* 1989;71B:851-855.

34. Murray WR: Use of antibiotic-containing bone cement. *Clin Orthop* 1984;190:89-95.

35. Elson RA: Exchange arthroplasty for infection: Perspectives from the United Kingdom. *Orthop Clin North Am* 1993;24:761-767.

36. Salvati EA, Chekofsky KM, Brause BD, Wilson PD Jr: Reimplantation in infection: A 12-year experience. *Clin Orthop* 1982;170:62-75.

37. Garvin KL, Evans BG, Salvati EA, Brause BD: Palacos gentamicin for the treatment of deep periprosthetic hip infections. *Clin Orthop* 1994; 298:97-105.

38. Garvin KL, Hanssen AD: Infection after total hip arthroplasty: Past, present, and future. *J Bone Joint Surg* 1995;77A:1576-1588.

SPECIAL CONSIDERATIONS

JOHN ANTONIOU, MD, PhD

REVISION FOR INSTABILITY

Dislocation is now the most common complication following total hip arthroplasty. In the case of primary arthroplasty, the rate has been reported at 2% to 5%.[1-5] The dislocation rate for revision arthroplasty has been reported at up to 20%.[5-6] There have been some reports of dislocation rates as low as 0.4%, but these centers represent the exception rather than the rule.[7] Dislocation rates also seem to diminish with increased time after the surgical intervention.[5] The latter may be due to the formation of a fibrous pseudocapsule and improvement in muscle tone. Despite these, dislocations can still occur many years after surgery.

Several studies have attempted to identify preoperative predisposing factors that result in an increased risk of dislocation. The patient's sex has been identified as a significant risk factor. The female to male ratio for dislocation has been documented at 2:1 in several series.[8,9] In dislocations occurring over 5 years after surgery, the rate increases to almost 3:1.[10] Medical conditions such as neuromuscular conditions and mental confusion have been associated with increased dislocation rates (22% to 75% of patients with one or more dislocations have an associated condition of the aforementioned kind).[2] Previous hip surgery is a predisposing factor for dislocation, with rates ranging from 4.8% to 33%.[2,9,11,12] The surgeon's experience also has been identified as an important contributing factor. Although most studies have noted this trend accidentally, a Swedish hip registry study clearly has demonstrated that inexperienced surgeons had over twice the dislocation rate.[13] In addition, the rate was inversely related to the number of arthroplasties performed. The most controversial predisposing factor to dislocation is surgical approach. Several studies have not demonstrated a statistically different rate between anterolateral, direct lateral, and posterior approaches.[1,13,14] However, some studies have determined that approach represents a major predisposing factor with the anterolateral approach associated with a lower dislocation rate than the posterior approach.[9,15,16] This issue remains a point of contention, and it is difficult to draw any conclusions from the available literature.

Some component design features have been associated with a decreased risk of dislocation; for example, liner hoods have been associated with a decreased dislocation rate in some studies. In a Mayo Clinic study, the dislocation rate decreased from 3.85% to 2.19%.[17] Unfortunately, the indiscriminate use of such components also increases the likelihood of impingement. In theory, femoral head size was believed to be an important variable in dislocation risk. In the clinical setting, this has never been shown to be statistically significant with femoral sizes in the 22 to 32 mm range.[1,9] The head to neck diameter ratio is an important variable in determining component range of motion before impingement and dislocation.[18] This is an important consideration when determining which femoral head component to use. A collared femoral head has a higher neck diameter; therefore, a smaller range of motion is available prior to impingement and subsequent dislocation. Femoral offset also has been shown to be an important variable in postoperative dislocation.[2] An increased femoral offset diminishes the chance of trochanteric impingement and increases abductor and soft-tissue tension.

Regardless of the preoperative risk, a dislocated total hip arthroplasty requires an immediate assessment of cause. Causal mechanisms associated with dislocations include component-anatomic impingement, component malposition, soft-tissue tension (including abductor muscles), and noncompliance.

Impingement can be due to bone, soft tissue, or the implant itself. A fulcrum is created by one of these structures and results in the dislocation of the implant. It is important to evaluate the possibility of bone and soft-tissue impingement at the time of surgery given that it is easily avoidable. As mentioned earlier, the femoral component can impinge on part of the acetabulum. This impingement can be caused by a diminished head to neck diameter ratio, impingement on a hooded liner, or a malpositioned implant, and it must be assessed at the time of revision surgery.

Component malposition is an important consideration in the patient with recurrent dislocation. Ali Khan and associates[1] demonstrated that almost half of the acetabular components were malpositioned in a review of 142 patients with hip dislocations. Ideally, the acetabular component should be placed in approximately 15° to 25° of anteversion and 40° of abduction. Although it never has been proven clinically, femoral component anteversion is undoubtedly an important consideration. In particular, the additive femoral and acetabular anteversion should be assessed (approximately 45° is ideal).

Soft-tissue tension is another variable that must be considered in the face of dislocation. Although difficult to assess clinically, causes of this condition include weakened abductors, muscle imbalance resulting from a neurologic deficit, deficient or nonunited trochanter, limb shortening, reduced femoral offset, and extensive soft-tissue dissection. Trochanteric nonunion has been associated with a 17.6% (with at least a 1-cm migration) to 28% dislocation rate.[9] Finally, a noncompliant patient who does not respect hip precautions can be the sole cause of multiple dislocations despite a perfectly placed component.

HIP DISLOCATION

Before reducing a hip arthroplasty dislocation, adequate anteroposterior (AP) and lateral radiographic assessment is required. Once the direction of the dislocation is determined, sedation is given and an attempted closed reduction is performed. In the case of anterior dislocation, in-line traction with internal rotation is required for reduction. A posterior dislocation can be treated using one of many reduction maneuvers that involve a variation of traction applied to a flexed and adducted hip. Despite adequate sedation and muscle relaxation, an open reduction is occasionally required (up to 10% of cases).[2]

Nonsurgical Treatment

In most instances, the treatment for a first-time dislocation is nonsurgical. Most surgeons prefer to use a hip brace that restricts motion and prevents redislocation. This initial restriction is supposed to allow for soft-tissue healing. Most braces allow for about 15° of abduction and 45° to 75° of flexion. The bracing period usually varies from 6 to 8 weeks up to 6 to 9 months. The results reported in the literature indicate a reasonable success rate for the first-time dislocation (80% to 100%)[19,20] but a high failure rate (approximately 60%) in recurrent dislocations.[20] Although some surgeons prefer the use of a spica cast because of the more secure limitation in mobility, many patients do not seem to tolerate this type of treatment. Use of bed rest or balanced suspension have not proven to be clearly superior to bracing and thus are not advocated.

Surgical Treatment

Of all types of revisions, revision for instability has traditionally been associated with the least satisfactory results.[21] Thus, a decision to perform a surgical intervention should not be taken lightly. Unless there is a clear technical reason, most dislocations that occur in the first few months are treated nonsurgically given that previous reports have indicated 60% of cases that dislocated in the first 5 weeks did not redislocate.[1] Any dislocation after this time frame was associated with a 40% successful nonsurgical treatment. Unfortunately, there is a diminished success rate associated with conservative treatment of a second dislocation and an even further diminished likelihood of success with three or more dislocations.

Once it is apparent that conservative measures will not work, surgical treatment should be considered. In general, 40% of patients will have malorientation of the components and the other 60% will have multiple variables to consider.[1,9] A preoperative plan that includes a detailed history should be formulated. A dislocation within 3 months is associated with soft-tissue factors (including diminished abductor tension) or impingement. After 3 months, dislocations are associated with component malposition or trochanteric insufficiency. After 5 years, there is a higher incidence of polyethylene wear.[10] The surgeon also should determine whether the hip is dislocated anteriorly or posteriorly. Radiographic assessment should include AP, a direct lateral, and frog-lateral views. These views will allow for assessing component orientation, femoral offset, possible sources of impingement, and integrity of the greater trochanter. If the cause is not obvious, some authors advocate assessment under fluoroscopy or aspiration of the hip if infection is suspected. Once a precise determination of the cause has been made, a directed procedure should be undertaken while preparing for all possibilities. In all, there are six corrective procedures (or a combination thereof) that can be undertaken. These include reorienting the component, augmenting soft-tissue and abductor tension, removing sources of impingement, exchanging of a worn liner, using constrained liners, and the Girdlestone procedure. Despite this extensive preoperative planning, surgical intervention for instability has not been very successful. The Mayo Clinic experience has indicated that in 95 surgical procedures, 70% success was achieved when there was a clearly identifiable reason for dislocation (mostly malposition).[22] If the cause of the instability was unclear or if removal of impingement was the only procedure, the success rate fell to less than 50%.

COMPONENT REORIENTATION

As mentioned previously, acetabular malposition is more common than femoral malposition. In the case of modular components, the surgeon has the choice of using a hooded liner or revising the entire acetabular component. With nonmodular components, the entire component usually is revised. The use of elevated rim liners does not increase the safe arc of motion; rather, it reorients it according to the position of the elevation.[23] Acetabular component reorientation is an easier undertaking than femoral component revision; thus, in mild cases of femoral version problems, some surgeons prefer to compensate on the acetabular side.

AUGMENTING SOFT-TISSUE AND ABDUCTOR TENSION

There are various options to consider when contemplating soft-tissue augmentation. These include greater trochanter advancement, increasing the femoral offset, increasing femoral neck length, more proximal placement of a new component, or moving the center of rotation lateral or distal. The decision to use one technique over another depends on whether the length of the affected leg is equal or longer, whether components are well ingrown and appropriately positioned, and whether placing a longer femoral head would require using a skirted component (which would increase the likelihood of impingement). If all of these conditions are true, then the surgeon would be more inclined to perform a greater trochanteric advancement. This procedure has been associated with variable results. Fraser and Wroblewski[6] have reported a 20% failure rate, whereas Ekelund[24] demonstrated two failures in 21 cases, and Kaplan and associates[25] revealed a 19% redislocation rate.

Removing Sources of Impingement

As mentioned earlier, impingement can be caused by bone, soft tissue, or the implant itself.

Preoperative or intraoperative assessment is necessary to identify any one of these conditions. It is always important to keep in mind that any surgical intervention only addressing treatment of impingement will result in a lower success rate (< 50%).[22]

Constrained Liners

Use of constrained liners has gained popularity because of the dismal results associated with procedures performed in cases where there is no clear causal mechanism. This is also a popular procedure in patients who are low demand and who cannot medically tolerate an extensive procedure, patients with severe soft-tissue or abductor dysfunction, or patients with failed previous surgical intervention for instability. The downside of these implants is that they limit the range of motion slightly, they transfer the dislocating torque to the implant-bone interface thus increasing the likelihood of early implant loosening, and an open reduction is required if there is ever a dislocation with one of these implants in place.

The amount of force that is transferred to the implant-bone interface depends on the amount of constraint provided by the implant. There have been a few reports on various constrained liner designs. The S-ROM design (Johnson & Johnson, Stamford, CT) is a constrained polyethylene liner with a locking ring that is screw locked to the underlying socket. Lombardi and associates[26] reported on five failures in 57 implants at 24 to 37 months, while Anderson and associates[27] reported six failures in 21 implants at 24 to 64 months. Two of these 11 failures were associated with an implant-bone interface loosening. The Osteonics design (Osteonics, Allendale, NJ) is a constrained tripolar device. Goetz and associates[28] have reported on 55 revisions at average 64 months with only two failures (96% success). The DePuy design (DePuy, Warsaw, IN) is a constrained polyethylene liner with a locking ring that is snap fit to the underlying socket. In a review of my patients, I examined 64 constrained liners at 3.8 years (three types, S-ROM, Osteonics, and DePuy). Twelve (16%) of the components were revised at a mean of 1.4 years (± 1.2 years; range 0.1 to 3.3). Seven (9.5%) of the components redislocated, one failed as a result of a mismatched liner cup dissociation, one failed because of a malpositioned cup, one failed because of cage failure, and two constructs resulted in implant-bone interface loosening. No type of liner was significantly worse than the others. There was no radiographic evidence of eccentric wear or periprosthetic osteolysis. These results are reasonable given the alternative of continued dislocation. Despite these results, use of these implants continues to be experimental and the surgeon must be wary of the long-term implications.

REVISION FOR PERIPROSTHETIC FRACTURE

Periprosthetic fractures can represent a difficult dilemma. The incidence of these fractures varies depending on implant technique and whether they occur before or after surgery. The incidence of perioperative fractures in primary cemented stems is less than 1%, whereas that of cementless stems varies from 3% to 20%.[29-32] The incidence of perioperative fractures in cemented revisions varies from 3% to 6.3%[33,34] and that in cementless revisions can be as high as 46%.[29] Postoperative fracture rates are not as well characterized but it is generally accepted that the incidence is higher in revision cases than it is in primary arthroplasty.

Many classification techniques have been described. The most important question to be answered when assessing a periprosthetic fracture is whether or not the implant is stable. Other variables to consider include bone quality, fracture pattern, fracture level, and patient's health and functional goals. Johansson and associates[35] described the fractures relative to their location. Type I fractures are proximal to the tip, type II fractures are located around the tip of the stem, and type III are located entirely distal to the stem. Subsequent classification systems not only have described the location of the fracture but also the stability of the implant and the quality of the bone stock[30,36-38] (Fig. 1).

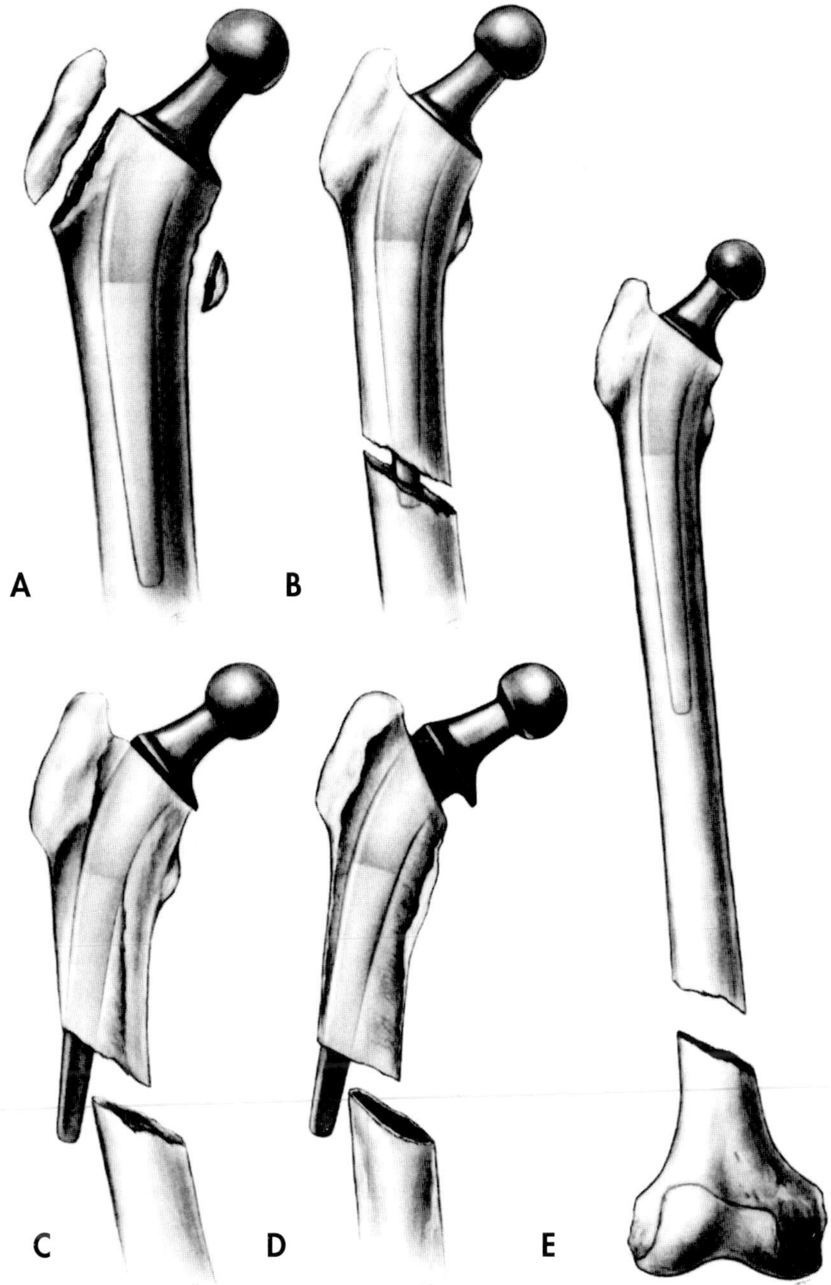

FIGURE 1
Vancouver classification of periprosthetic fractures. **A,** Type A involves the greater or lesser trochanter. **B,** Type B1 is a stable fracture around the stem. **C,** Type B2 is an unstable fracture around a stem. **D,** Type B3 is an unstable fracture around a stem associated with significant diaphyseal bone loss. **E,** Type C is a fracture distal to the stem. (Reproduced with permission from Garbuz, DS, Masri BA, Duncan CP: Fractures of the femur, in Steinberg ME, Garino JP (eds): *Revision Total Hip Arthroplasty.* Philadelphia, PA, Lippincott-Williams & Wilkins, 1999, pp 493-503.)

NONSURGICAL TREATMENT

Nonsurgical treatment includes the spectrum of limited weight bearing, spica cast, and/or cast brace to skeletal traction. Limited weight bearing is reserved for stable fractures around a stable implant, usually a perioperative longitudinal fracture involving the proximal femur that was suffered while inserting a cementless stem. Other fracture management depends on fracture stability and patient compliance.

There have been several studies on the results of nonsurgical treatment.[35,39,40] Although there is an increased nonunion rate, healing can be achieved. However, many complications are associated with this kind of intervention. Treatment such as traction, spica cast, and prolonged bed rest can result in complications including skin ulcers, fat embolism, and pneumonia. Even with healing of the fracture, there is an increased risk of malunion, delayed union, and early prosthetic loosening.

Despite these risks, there are some indications for nonsurgical treatment of periprosthetic fractures. A minimally displaced fracture around a stable implant can be treated with restricted weight bearing. Considerations in deciding to treat an implant nonsurgically include alignment that can be maintained with nonsurgical measures, a stable implant, and a fracture located in the proximal or middle regions of the implant with adequate stability being provided by a stable implant. The surgeon must always keep in mind that fractures at the tip of the implant are associated with a 25% to 42% nonunion rate when treated nonsurgically.[36] This is in stark contrast to the 90% to 100% success rate noted after surgical intervention.[36-38]

SURGICAL TREATMENT

Given the morbidity associated with nonsurgical treatment, secure fixation is preferred in order to allow early patient mobilization. The most clear indications for surgical treatment include a loose or broken prosthesis, the inability to obtain or maintain adequate alignment, or a fracture that extends distal to the tip of the prosthesis.

The surgical options include extramedullary fixation, intramedullary fixation, revision of the femoral component to a longer stem, or a combination of the above. The type of fixation required depends on the fracture pattern and whether the implant is loose.

If the implant is loose and there is still over 4 cm of intact diaphysis remaining (some recommend a bypass by at least twice the bone diameter), the most obvious option is to revise the stem to a long fully porous-coated stem that takes advantage of bypass fixation. If there is significant proximal bone loss with this type of fracture, femoral bone stock can be augmented by using a strut allograft. When a prosthesis is used in this situation, the combined refracture, nonunion, and revision rates are in the vicinity of 12% to 20%.[37] If the implant is loose and the diaphysis is compromised, implant revision to a longer component is still advised. If stability of this implant is still in question once it is inserted, the fixation may be augmented by extramedullary fixation, including Dall-Miles plates or strut and cerclage fixation. If a significant amount of proximal bone loss is present, the surgeon should consider a proximal femoral replacement in the elderly patient and an allograft prosthetic composite in the younger patient. The surgeon should bear in mind that the later two options are still considered experimental, with no long-term results available. It is generally accepted that loose-stem revision should be performed with a cementless component. In the periprosthetic fracture setting, cemented revisions have been noted to perform much less well than cementless revisions.[39]

In the case of periprosthetic fractures associated with a stable implant, extramedullary or intramedullary fixation can be considered (Fig. 2). The extramedullary techniques that have been reported on include AO plate and screw fixation, cerclage wire fixation, cortical bone and cerclage wiring, and Parnham bands with Ogden plate or Dall-Miles plate fixation. Fracture union rates from 90% to 100% have been reported but complications, such as fracture below the plate, nonunion, and component loosening, as high as 80% also have been reported.[37,38,41] Cerclage wiring alone has been associated with a lower success rate than cerclage wiring associated with a longitudinal fixation.[42] There has been a recent advent of intramedullary fixation for

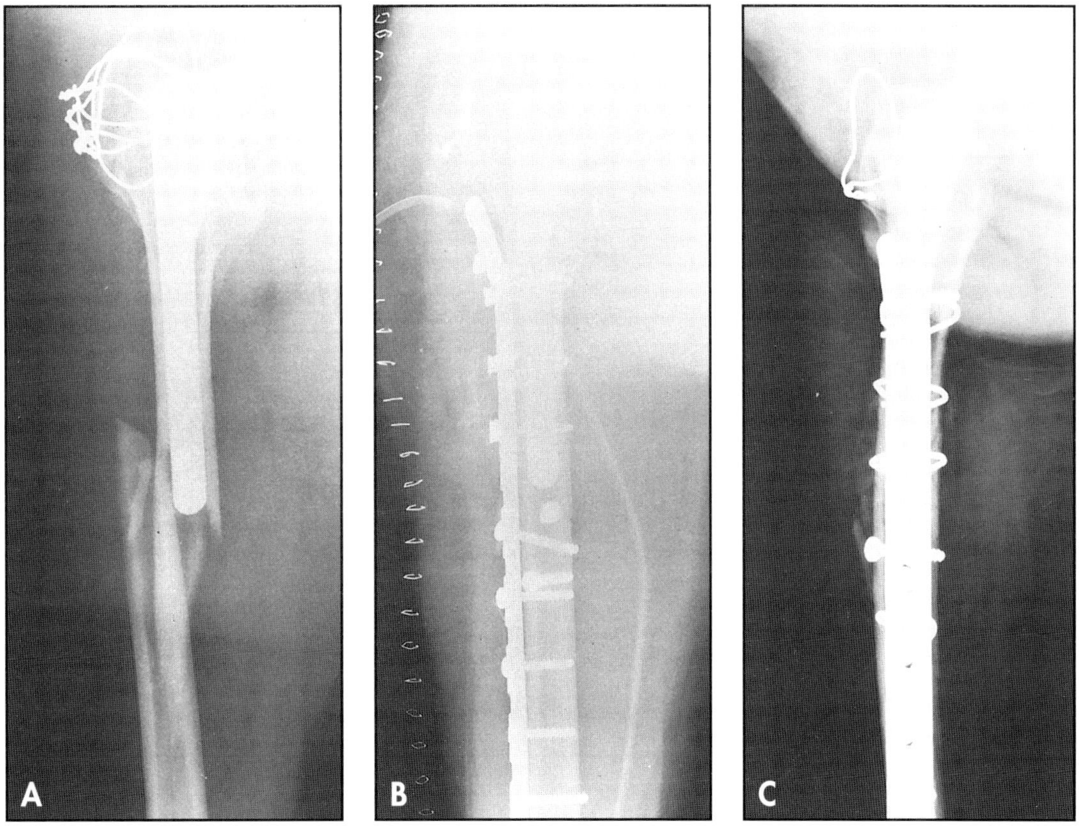

FIGURE 2
A 42-year-old man with a stable periprosthetic fracture around an uncemented stem. This implant was successfully treated with a modified plate for screw and cerclage fixation. (Reproduced with permission from Kelley SS: Periprosthetic femoral fractures. *J Am Acad Orthop Surg* 1994;2:164-172.)

periprosthetic fractures associated with a stable implant. This technique involves the use of trephine components that are custom fit to be impacted or cemented to the distal tip of the femoral component. When performing this technique, the surgeon must be careful not to destabilize the component proximally. Once the trephine is fixed to the component, a distal extension is impacted down the femoral canal. The two segments are joined at a Morse taper junction. Such custom intramedullary fixation is relatively new, and no long-term clinical results are available.

The biggest controversy as to the type of treatment required concerns the midregion periprosthetic fracture around a well-fixed component. In the case of noncomminuted fractures in which good stability is provided by the implant, nonsurgical treatment is appropriate. If there is any comminution present, surgical treatment is indicated. Unfortunately, open reduction and plate fixation has been associated with a nonunion and refracture rate from 10% to 80%.[38,41] Thus, a periprosthetic fracture in which there is any question of implant stability, including increased comminution, should be treated with revision of the stem to a fully porous-coated implant. This treatment should be case specific, and part of the decision is made intraoperatively.

In the case of periprosthetic fracture with associated septic loosening, there are no long-term clinical studies available on which to base treatment. Despite this lack, it is generally agreed that the first goal of treatment is fracture stabilization. Thus, infections should be managed by removing

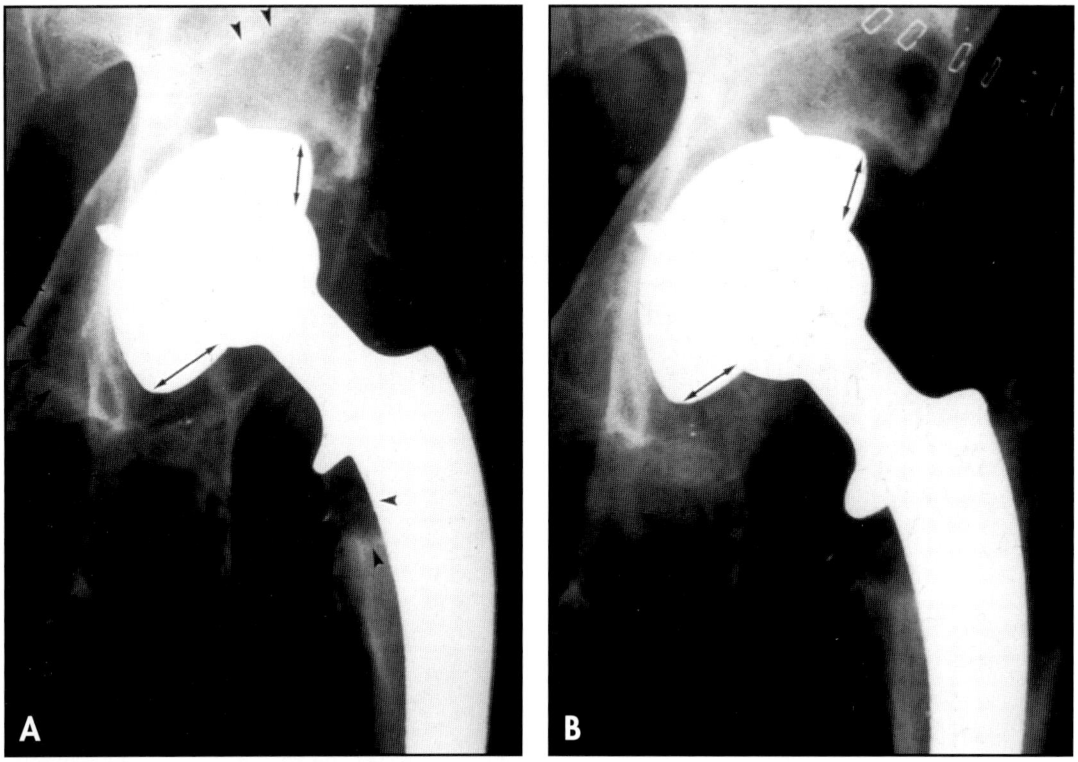

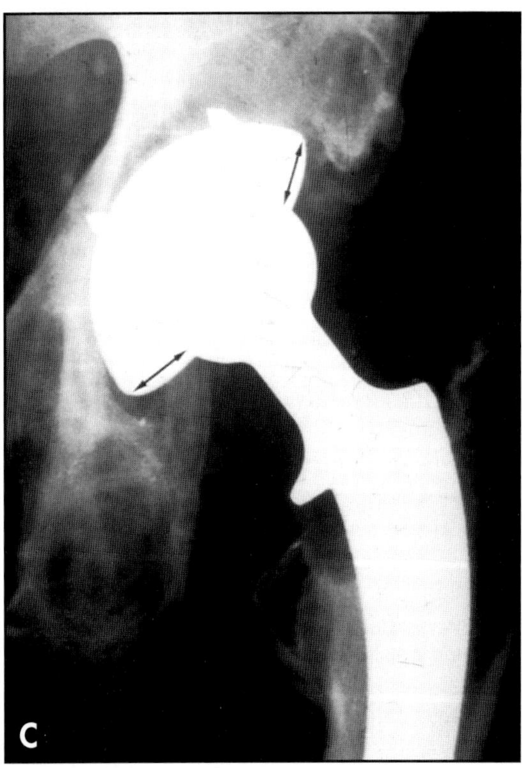

FIGURE 3
A, Severe ischial and ileum osteolysis secondary to polyethylene wear. **B,** Postoperative polyethylene liner exchange and grafting of osteolytic defect in ischium and ileum with cancellous bone. **C,** Resolution of osteolysis at 2.5 year postliner exchange and bone grafting.

the loose prosthesis, debriding the necrotic tissue, and stabilizing the fracture. It is not yet clear whether implantation of the new prosthesis should be performed immediately or in two stages, or whether cemented or cementless components should be used.

REVISION FOR ISOLATED PROGRESSIVE OSTEOLYSIS

Osteolysis has been attributed to the reaction of bone to wear debris. As the duration of follow-up studies increase, the frequency of this event in the femur and acetabulum has increased.[43-47] The patterns of periprosthetic osteolysis in the pelvis differ depending on whether the acetabular component was inserted with or without cement.[48] With cemented sockets, periprosthetic bone resorption frequently occurs in a linear fashion. Osteolysis surrounding a well-fixed porous-coated acetabular component inserted without cement is usually an isolated expansile lesion. Because of the localized nature of the osteolysis, the implant is not usually loosened despite an extensive destruction of bone. Thus, there can be a great deal of bone loss before the patient becomes symptomatic and before the diagnosis is made. Traditionally, the surgical approach to this problem was to remove the acetabular component, fill the lesion in the pelvis with bone graft, and insert a new component.

Removal of a stable component often leads to further destruction of the acetabular bone stock, compromising the subsequent reconstruction. Such an intervention can result in a defect of the medial wall of the acetabulum, in severe damage to the anterior and posterior columns, or in pelvic discontinuity.

In the case of a stable acetabular component, the trend now is to exchange the acetabular liner, debride the osteolytic lesion, and pack the osteolytic lesion with allograft bone chips.[49] First-generation porous-coated acetabular components resulted in a high incidence of osteolytic lesions. Schmalzried and associates[46] described pelvic osteolysis in 17% of 113 hips with a porous-coated cementless titanium acetabular shell. Maloney and associates[44] described 14 patients who had pelvic osteolysis in cementless porous-coated acetabular shells. The mean time to presentation was 65 months. All but one of the sockets were stable, and 11 of the 14 patients had a Harris Hip Score of more than 90 points.

Maloney and associates[49] reported on 35 patients who underwent a revision procedure to treat pelvic osteolysis surrounding stable cementless porous-coated acetabular components. The procedure included acetabular liner exchange, the debridement of osteolytic lesion, and packing of the lesion with allograft bone chips (Fig. 3). The size of the 46 distinct pelvic osteolytic lesions noted around the 35 cups ranged from 0.5 × 0.5 cm to 6.3 × 2.7 cm (mean, 2.6 × 1.7 cm). At the time of identification, 35 patients had no or only slight occasional pain in the hip, emphasizing the need for vigilant postoperative surveillance of patients who have had a total hip arthroplasty. Seventeen of 21 patients who had pain before the revision had identifiable mechanical causes of pain, unrelated to the periacetabular osteolysis. The remaining four patients had evidence of marked synovitis of the hip. The patients were evaluated a minimum of 2 years (range, 2 to 5 years; mean, 3.3 years) after the revision operation. In all cases, the sockets were found to be stable, the bone grafts appeared nicely integrated, and there was no evidence of progression of the osteolytic defects. One third of the lesions were no longer visible on radiographs, and the remaining two thirds had decreased in size.

Some believe that complete debridement of the granuloma is essential in stopping the osteolysis. Others argue that sustained particle load is required to drive the osteolytic process. It is largely believed that the replacement of the liner would eliminate the source of the high particle load. In this study, liner replacement proved to be more important than complete removal of the granuloma given that none of the osteolytic defects continued to enlarge after the revision and that one third of the lesions resolved completely even if they had not been filled with bone graft.[49]

Thus, in the face of a stable acetabular component with a periacetabular osteolytic defect, exchange of the liner and debridement of the granuloma, with or without use of bone chips, is a reasonable alternative to revision of the socket. Of course, the locking mechanism must be intact for this procedure to work. If the locking mechanism is deficient, the component should be revised or cementing the liner into the acetabular shell may be an option in some low-demand patients. In addition, the acetabular shell must be large enough to allow for a 6-mm thick polyethylene liner.

REFERENCES

1. Ali Khan MA, Brakenbury PH, Reynolds IS: Dislocation following total hip replacement. *J Bone Joint Surg* 1981;63B:214-218.
2. Fackler CD, Poss R: Dislocation in total hip arthroplasties. *Clin Orthop* 1980;151:169-178.
3. Hedlundh U, Ahnfelt L, Fredin H: Incidence of dislocation after hip arthroplasty: Comparison of different registration methods in 408 cases. *Acta Orthop Scand* 1992;63:403-406.
4. Lindberg HO, Carlsson AS, Gentz CF, Pettersson H: Recurrent and non-recurrent dislocation following total hip arthroplasty. *Acta Orthop Scand* 1982;53:947-952.
5. Morrey BF: Instability after total hip arthroplasty. *Orthop Clin North Am* 1992;23:237-248.
6. Fraser GA, Wroblewski BM: Revision of the Charnley low-friction arthroplasty for recurrent or irreducible dislocation. *J Bone Joint Surg* 1981;63B:552-555.
7. Etienne A, Cupic Z, Charnley J: Postoperative dislocation after Charnley low-friction arthroplasty. *Clin Orthop* 1978;132:19-23.
8. Khan MT, Stockley I, Ibbotson C: Allograft bone transplantation: A Sheffield experience. *Ann R Coll Surg Engl* 1998;80:150-153.
9. Woo RY, Morrey BF: Dislocations after total hip arthroplasty. *J Bone Joint Surg* 1982;64A:1295-1306.
10. Coventry MB: Late dislocations in patients with Charnley total hip arthroplasty. *J Bone Joint Surg* 1985;67A:832-841.
11. Possai KW, Dorr LD, McPherson EJ: Metal ring supports for deficient acetabular bone in total hip replacement, in Pritchard DJ (ed): *Instructional Course Lectures 45*. Rosemont, IL, American Academy of Orthopaedic Surgeons, 1996, pp 161-169.
12. Williams JF, Gottesman MJ, Mallory TH: Dislocation after total hip arthroplasty: Treatment with an above-knee hip spica cast. *Clin Orthop* 1982;171:53-58.
13. Hedlundh U, Hybbinette CH, Fredin H: Influence of surgical approach on dislocations after Charnley hip arthroplasty. *J Arthroplasty* 1995;10:609-614.
14. Pace TB: Total hip arthroplasty: Are early dislocations related to surgical approach. *J Orthop Tech* 1994;2:173-176.
15. Roberts JM, Fu FH, McClain EJ, Ferguson AB Jr: A comparison of the posterolateral and anterolateral approaches to total hip arthroplasty. *Clin Orthop* 1984;187:205-210.
16. Robinson RP, Robinson HJ Jr, Salvati EA: Comparison of the transtrochanteric and posterior approaches for total hip replacement. *Clin Orthop* 1980;147:143-147.
17. Cobb TK, Morrey BF, Ilstrup DM: The elevated-rim acetabular liner in total hip arthroplasty: Relationship to postoperative dislocation. *J Bone Joint Surg* 1996;78A:80-86.
18. Amstutz HC, Lodwig RM, Schurman DJ, Hodgson AG: Range of motion studies for total hip replacements: A comparative study with a new experimental apparatus. *Clin Orthop* 1975;111:124-130.
19. Dorr LD, Wolf AW, Chandler R, Conaty JP: Classification and treatment of dislocations of total hip arthroplasty. *Clin Orthop* 1983;173:151-158.
20. Stewart HD: The hip cast-brace for hip prosthesis instability. *Ann R Coll Surg Engl* 1983;65:404-406.
21. Kavanagh BF, Ilstrup DM, Fitzgerald RH Jr: Revision total hip arthroplasty. *J Bone Joint Surg* 1985;67A:517-526.
22. Daly PJ, Morrey BF: Operative correction of an unstable total hip arthroplasty. *J Bone Joint Surg* 1992;74A:1334-1343.

23. Krushell RJ, Burke DW, Harris WH: Elevated-rim acetabular components: Effect on range of motion and stability in total hip arthroplasty. *J Arthroplasty* 1991;6(suppl 1):S53-S58.

24. Ekelund A: Trochanteric osteotomy for recurrent dislocation of total hip arthroplasty. *J Arthroplasty* 1993;8:629-632.

25. Kaplan SJ, Thomas WH, Poss R: Trochanteric advancement for recurrent dislocation after total hip arthroplasty. *J Arthroplasty* 1987;2:119-124.

26. Lombardi AV Jr, Mallory TH, Kraus TJ, Vaughn BK: Preliminary report on the S-ROM constraining acetabular insert: A retrospective clinical experience. *Orthopedics* 1991;14:297-303.

27. Anderson MJ, Murray WR, Skinner HB: Constrained acetabular components. *J Arthroplasty* 1994;9:17-23.

28. Goetz DD, Capello WN, Callaghan JJ, Brown TD, et al: Salvage of a recurrently dislocating total hip prosthesis with use of a constrained acetabular component: A retrospective analysis of fifty-six cases. *J Bone Joint Surg* 1998;80A:502-509.

29. Fitzgerald RH Jr, Brindley GW, Kavanagh BF: The uncemented total hip arthroplasty: Intraoperative femoral fractures. *Clin Orthop* 1988; 235:61-66.

30. Schwartz JT Jr, Mayer JG, Engh CA: Femoral fracture during non-cemented total hip arthroplasty. *J Bone Joint Surg* 1989;71A:1135-1142.

31. Scott RD, Turner RH, Leitzes SM, Aufranc OE: Femoral fractures in conjunction with total hip replacement. *J Bone Joint Surg* 1975;57A:494-501.

32. Stuchin SA: Femoral shaft fracture in porous and press-fit total hip arthroplasty. *Orthop Rev* 1990;19:153-159.

33. Christensen CM, Seger BM, Schultz RB: Management of intraoperative femur fractures associated with revision hip arthroplasty. *Clin Orthop* 1989;248:177-180.

34. Kavanagh BF: Femoral fractures associated with total hip arthroplasty. *Orthop Clin North Am* 1992;23:249-257.

35. Johansson JE, McBroom R, Barrington TW, Hunter GA: Fracture of the ipsilateral femur in patients with total hip replacement. *J Bone Joint Surg* 1981;63A:1435-1442.

36. Bethea JS III, DeAndrade JR, Fleming LL, Lindenbaum SD, Welch RB: Proximal femoral fractures following total hip arthroplasty. *Clin Orthop* 1982;170:95-106.

37. Cooke PH, Newman JH: Fractures of the femur in relation to cemented hip prostheses. *J Bone Joint Surg* 1988;70B:386-389.

38. Serocki JH, Chandler RW, Dorr LD: Treatment of fractures about hip prostheses with compression plating. *J Arthroplasty* 1992;7:129-135.

39. Beals RK, Tower SS: Periprosthetic fractures of the femur: An analysis of 93 fractures. *Clin Orthop* 1996;327:238-246.

40. Jensen JS, Barfod G, Hansen D, et al: Femoral shaft fracture after hip arthroplasty. *Acta Orthop Scand* 1988;59:9-13.

41. Zenni EJ Jr, Pomeroy DL, Caudle RJ: Ogden plate and other fixations for fractures complicating femoral endoprostheses. *Clin Orthop* 1988;231:83-90.

42. Partridge AJ, Evans PE: The treatment of fractures of the shaft of the femur using nylon cerclage. *J Bone Joint Surg* 1982;64B:210-214.

43. Maloney WJ, Jasty M, Harris WH, Galante JO, Callaghan JJ: Endosteal erosion in association with stable uncemented femoral components. *J Bone Joint Surg* 1990;72A:1025-1034.

44. Maloney WJ, Peters P, Engh CA, Chandler H: Severe osteolysis of the pelvic in association with acetabular replacement without cement. *J Bone Joint Surg* 1993;75A:1627-1635.

45. Maloney WJ, Woolson ST: Increasing incidence of femoral osteolysis in association with uncemented Harris-Galante total hip arthroplasty: A follow-up report. *J Arthroplasty* 1996;11:130-134.

46. Schmalzried TP, Guttmann D, Grecula M, Amstutz HC: The relationship between the design, position, and articular wear of acetabular components inserted without cement and the development of pelvic osteolysis. *J Bone Joint Surg* 1994;76A:677-688.

47. Tanzer M, Maloney WJ, Jasty M, Harris WH: The progression of femoral cortical osteolysis in association with total hip arthroplasty without cement. *J Bone Joint Surg* 1992;74A:404-410.

48. Zicat B, Engh CA, Gokcen E: Patterns of osteolysis around total hip components inserted with and without cement. *J Bone Joint Surg* 1995; 77A:432-439.

49. Maloney WJ, Herzwurm P, Paprosky W, Rubash HE, Engh CA: Treatment of pelvic osteolysis associated with a stable acetabular component inserted without cement as part of a total hip replacement. *J Bone Joint Surg* 1997; 79A:1628-1634.

COMPLICATIONS OF REVISION TOTAL HIP ARTHROPLASTY

NELSON GREIDANUS, MD, MPH

INTRAOPERATIVE COMPLICATIONS

Revision total hip arthroplasty is a complex surgical procedure that requires great expertise. A surgeon performing revision total hip arthroplasty must have the proper training and experience to successfully execute such a difficult procedure and achieve a successful outcome. Although many complications have been reported during primary total hip arthroplasty, these and other complications are encountered more frequently and with higher degrees of severity during revision total hip arthroplasty. The time required for completion of the procedure, the amount of bleeding, and the degree of osteoporosis and osteolysis are related to some of the complications. Other causes, including preexisting health problems such as congestive heart failure, asthma, diabetes, hypertension, and systemic arthritis involving other joints, have been identified.

The best single defense against complications is adequate preparation. All patients should undergo a comprehensive preoperative history and physical assessment. To minimize surgical time and blood loss, preoperative planning should anticipate all equipment needed and approximate length of time of the procedure. The surgeon should ensure that adequate blood products and cell saver systems are available.

Intraoperative monitoring should include an indwelling urinary catheter and arterial lines if the anesthesiologist desires them. The patient should be positioned to minimize pressure on the axilla, which could give rise to a brachial plexus palsy. Pressure points should be padded to avoid pressure-related nerve problems and skin breakdown. Care must be taken to protect other delicate joint replacements or skeletal problems that may go awry during positioning.

INFECTION

Although infection usually manifests itself during the postoperative period, contamination usually occurs during the surgical procedure. Operating room personnel must practice aseptic technique with respect to the patient, operating room, instruments, and themselves. Perioperative antibiotic prophylaxis remains the single best method of preventing sepsis. The use of laminar flow, body exhaust suits, and ultraviolet light may also assist in maintaining a sterile field for surgery. Infection following revision total hip arthroplasty is more frequent than after a primary total hip replacement and is associated with considerable morbidity and mortality and a high cost of treatment. Predisposing risk factors include multiple previous hip surgeries, previous open reduction and internal fixation of acetabular fracture, previous hip infections, diabetes mellitus, inflammatory arthropathy, and collagen vascular disorders.

The most common presenting symptom in patients with an infected total hip arthroplasty is persistent pain. Pain that has not resolved since the operation or pain at rest are ominous symptoms of an inflammatory process that may be consistent with deep infection. The second most common sign of an infected total hip is persistent drainage. If suspicious, the surgeon should not hesitate to obtain a thorough history and physical examination in addition to obtaining a complete blood count with differential and C-reactive protein or erythrocyte sedimentation rate. The surgeon should not hesitate to perform a surgical debridement or exploration of a persistent draining wound.

The treatment of suprafascial subcutaneous wound infections follows the principles of treatment of all surgical wounds. Recovery of the organisms and the establishment of effective antibiotic treatment is of primary importance. Adequate drainage to evacuate loculated hematomas or abscesses is essential and permits culturing of fluids and tissues. Deep infection must be surgically drained in the acute postoperative period, and with aggressive debridement and antibiotics the prosthesis might possibly be spared from chronic infection. Gustilo and Tsukayama[1] reported 74% success in patients with an early postoperative infection, but only 50% in patients with an acute hematogenous infection.

BLEEDING

An important component of the preoperative assessment is obtaining a coagulation profile and hemoglobin levels. The surgeon and anesthesiologist must work together to minimize blood loss and maintain optimal hemodynamic status. Hypotensive anesthesia, meticulous hemostasis, and appropriate use of blood products and cell savers likely will result in an optimal result. Cell savers should not be used in the context of infected hip revision surgery. In further efforts to normalize the coagulation cascade, preoperative patient counseling should encourage patients to discontinue aspirin and nonsteroidal anti-inflammatory drugs if agreeable with the patient and internist.

VASCULAR INJURY

Intraoperative vascular injuries during total hip arthroplasty have been reported in many orthopaedic studies and occur more often in revision total hip arthroplasty. Intrapelvic vascular injuries can arise as a result of acetabular component or intrapelvic cement removal, the insertion of screws into the acetabulum or pelvis when reconstructing the acetabulum in the region of the sciatic notch, or if cement escapes and coagulates vessels while curing. Inadvertent injury to the femoral vessels can result from improper placement of the anterior Hohmann acetabular retractor or when securing distal femoral cerclage cables around femoral allograft. Shoenfeld and associates[2] reviewed the literature and found 68 cases and reported on five new cases of vascular injuries during hip arthroplasty, with 39% of cases occurring during revision procedures. Complications were related to incorporation of the iliac vessels in cement, aggressive medial retraction, excessive traction on the atherosclerotic vessel, and improper technique in preparation of the acetabulum. The most commonly injured vessels were the external iliac artery, femoral artery, and iliac vein. The mortality rate was 7% with a 15% incidence of limb loss.

Other vascular complications include embolic phenomena. Component insertion, and particularly cemented femoral insertion, results in a bolus of echogenic material that is delivered to the cardiopulmonary system and has given rise to the clinical picture of pulmonary embolism, hypotension, cardiac arrest, and death. Some authors support venting of the femoral canal in conjunction with plugging to avoid compression of the marrow.[3]

Deep venous thrombosis is a well-documented complication of primary and revision hip arthroplasty. Sharrock and associates[4] have determined that longer surgical procedures and the type of anesthesia administered influence the rate of deep venous thrombosis after total hip arthroplasty. Other systemic factors, such as a hypercoagulable state, obesity, immobility, and chronic illnesses also increase risk for deep venous thrombosis.

NEUROLOGIC COMPLICATIONS

Peripheral neurologic injury is a troublesome complication in revision hip arthroplasty. A review of the literature revealed an incidence ranging from 0.9% to 5.9% in primary arthroplasty and 2% to 7.6% in revision total hip arthroplasty.[5] The peroneal branch of the sciatic nerve was most commonly involved. Whereas minor stretch injury may have a spontaneous recovery, prolonged traction or traumatic compression of the nerve at the hip level may have a less favorable prognosis. Revision or reoperation requires prolonged and repeated retraction, especially along the posterior acetabulum for exposure. The literature suggests a high predisposition among women for sustaining nerve injury, with 79% of nerve injuries in one series being in female patients.[6] Other etiologic factors in sciatic nerve injury include cement polymerization, paralysis caused by bleeding and hematoma formation, entrapment of the sciatic nerve by wire during reattachment of the trochanter, and migration of trochanteric wires. Edwards and associates[7] have indicated that in 23 of their patients with palsies, an average limb lengthening of 2.7 cm may have contributed to peroneal nerve injury, while an average lengthening of 4.4 cm may lead to sciatic nerve injury.

LIMB-LENGTH INEQUALITY

Whereas the revision setting makes it more difficult for the surgeon to obtain perfectly symmetrical limb lengths, preoperative templating and appropriate component inventory may minimize this complication. Taller people tend to notice discrepancy less often than shorter people. It is important to discuss the possibility of limb-length inequality with patients before surgery.

HETEROTOPIC OSSIFICATION

The incidence of heterotopic ossification is variable and ranges from 8% to 70% in various series.[5] Most cases are minimal although ankylosis can occur. The most widely associated risk factors include male gender and/or a positive history of hypertrophic osteoarthritis, a history of heterotopic ossification, diffuse idiopathic skeletal hyperostosis, active ankylosing spondylolitis, and Paget disease. High-risk patients should be identified and prophylactic treatments administered to prevent this complication. Efforts should be made on the part of the surgeon to minimize tissue trauma and to irrigate bone debris and hematoma at completion of the procedure. The most accepted method of preventing heterotopic ossification is a single 600 to 700 mrad dose of radiation administered in the first 2 postoperative days.[8] Alternatives include indomethacin; however, results have been very good with radiation. Radiation may cause a delay in porous ingrowth and cause an increased incidence of delayed union or nonunion of a trochanteric osteotomy.

FRACTURE AND PERFORATION OF BONE

Fractures of the femoral shaft have been reported in numerous studies.[9] These often are associated with severe osteoporosis or protrusio acetabuli. Although usually proximal, fractures can occur anywhere along the femur intraoperatively. Small longitudinal fractures that start at the proximal femur with insertion of cementless stem can be wired to prevent propogation. In the early postoperative period, weight bearing can cause fracture of the proximal femur as the result of hoop stresses. Difficult anatomic conditions require good exposure, which may further minimize the likelihood of developing intraoperative fracture.

Perforation of the femoral shaft has been reported by Talab and associates.[10] Risk factors for perforation include previous hip operations, revision total hip arthroplasty, dysplasia, osteoporosis, and poor exposure. If a perforation is identified intraoperatively at the tip of the stem, a longer prosthesis can be used to bypass the perforation.

HIP DISLOCATION

Although incidence of dislocation ranges from 1% to 2% in primary arthroplasty, it can range as high as 25% in revision arthroplasty. It most likely is caused by component malpositioning or laxity of the soft tissues around the hip. Care must be taken to re-tension the abductors appropriately. This step can be facilitated by choice of components and site of reattachment of the greater trochanter if osteotomized. Full stability testing should be carried out while the patient is still under anesthesia because sources of impingement should be worked out while the patient is still on the operating table. Some surgeons select to routinely restrict the range of motion in revision hip arthroplasties for the first 6 weeks postoperatively in the hope of providing time for hip capsular healing and the return of normal muscle tone before challenging the limits of range of motion.

REFERENCES

1. Gustilo R, Tsukayama D: Treatment of infected cemented total hip arthroplasty with tobramycin beads and delayed revision with a cementless prosthesis and bone grafting. *Orthop Trans* 1988; 12:739.
2. Shoenfeld N, Stuchin S, Pearl R, Haveson S: The management of vascular injuries associated with total hip arthroplasty. *J Vas Surg* 1990;11: 549-555.
3. Wenda K, Degreif J, Rundel M, Ritter G: Pathogenesis and prophylaxis of circulatory reactions during total hip replacement. *Arch Orthop Trauma Surg* 1993;112:260-265.
4. Sharrock N, Ranawat C, Urquhart B, Peterson M: Factors influencing deep vein thrombosis following total hip arthroplasty under epidural anaesthesia. *Anesth Analg* 1993;76:765-771.
5. Nercessian O: Intraoperative complications, in Steinberg M (ed): *Revision Total Hip Arthroplasty,* New York, NY, Lippincott-Williams & Wilkins, 1999, pp 443-456.
6. Johanson N, Pellicci P, Tsairis P, Salvati E: Nerve injury in total hip arthroplasty. *Clin Orthop* 1983; 179:214.
7. Edwards B, Tullos H, Nobel P: Contributory factors and etiology of sciatic nerve palsy in total hip arthroplasty. *Clin Orthop* 1987;136:218.
8. Hedley A, Mead L, Hendren D: The prevention of heterotopic bone formation following total hip arthroplasty using 600 rad in a single dose. *J Arthroplasty* 1989;4:319-325.
9. Kavanagh B: Femoral fractures associated with total hip arthroplasty. *Orthop Clin North Am* 1992;23:249-257.
10. Talab Y, States J, Evarts C: Femoral shaft perforation: a complication of total hip reconstruction. *Clin Orthop* 1979;141:158-165.

INDEX